*"Before you heal someone,
ask him if he's willing to give up
the things that make him sick."*

— HIPPOCRATES

This book was produced in collaboration with Fearlesss
Literary Services, which represents all subsidiary rights.
Translation and republication inquiries can be
directed to *info@fearlessbooks.com*.

ISBN: 978-1-7335475-0-5

Library of Congress Control Number:
2018915203

COVER DESIGN
John Brenner
www.johnnyink.com

TYPOGRAPHY & INTERIOR DESIGN

D. Patrick Miller
Fearless Literary Services
www.fearlessbooks.com

AUTHOR PORTRAIT
Michelle Laurita

WTF* IS WRONG WITH OUR HEALTH?
(*What the Food)

A Rebel Physician's Manifesto for Reversing Disease and Increasing Smiles

by ROBERTO TOSTADO, MD

DEDICATION

To Amelie, my beautiful young wise daughter who is the reason for me being healthy, happy and smiling

INTRODUCTION

In some ways, it's disappointing that this book had to be written, because its starting point is the huge misfortune of health and health care in this current time. Everything I have to recommend in this book should already be taught at home, schools, and medical institutions. Knowing how to maintain optimum health with a sensible and enjoyable diet should be common sense, but too many people continue to feed their diseases and chronic discomfort instead. And they're encouraged by our medical system and massive pharmacological industry, which thrive on maintaining illness rather than preventing and healing it. Meanwhile the processed-food industry floods our supermarkets with denatured "foodstuffs," chock-full of sugar, toxins, and chemicals that weaken our bodies rather than nourish them.

This book is written for people who are tired of dieting to lose weight; for those who are sick of being told that their diabetes is a life sentence; and for those who are sick and tired of taking all kinds of medications every day for years, with no end in sight. This book is here to help you understand that your health is grounded on what you put in your body — and that food can be your medicine or your poison, depending on what you choose to eat every day.

This book is also for those who think a healthy diet sucks because it means eating cabbage and cauliflower all day long.

Not true! This book is also here to help you open your eyes, heart, mind, and mouth to the fact that a truly healthy diet is delicious and diverse.

I hope that you've judged this book by its cover, then opened it because you're ready to hear what I'm saying — something that many people may have felt for a while, but were perhaps reluctant to express out loud. We are in a moment that demands radical change, to preserve the health of our children and future generations through our choices. I can do all the talking, but actually doing what's necessary is completely on you. A friend of mine asked, "How can you make people want to be healthy?" My answer was simply that people have to know it's *possible* to be healthy without endless doctor visits and lifelong prescriptions. Then the healthy choice will be clear.

Finally, this book is for my colleagues in the medical community. More physicians are gaining a new understanding of real nutrition, as I did, and passing on this life-giving information to our patients. You can benefit greatly from this approach. I put in ten years of conventional practice with the Kaiser Permanente healthcare system in California, growing increasingly disenchanted as I began to question whether I was really helping people heal, or only providing assistance in the maintenance of their diseases. My anger and disappointment grew as I watched too many patients suffer heart attacks, even with normal cholesterol levels, and saw diabetics forced to suffer amputations despite increasing their insulin levels by the vials.

Finally, I'd had enough. For the last two years of my practice at Kaiser I focused on teaching health and wellness through lifestyle and food choices, and stopped focusing on drugs.

I attended a conference in San Diego sponsored by ACAM, the American College for Advancement in Medicine, where I found myself surrounded by physicians who expressed the same disgruntlement and frustrations, and wanted to make a difference through alternative approaches with creativity, conscientiousness and compassion. At this gathering of defiant fellow doctors, I learned that the fourth largest cause of death in this country was prescription drugs.[1] That was my light-bulb moment, when I realized we were licensed to heal but too often ended up killing instead; the statistics were undeniable. I wanted to quit medicine, and found myself at a crossroads, feeling lost and almost ashamed of my medical degree.

With the encouragement of my wife Teresa, whom I met during my residency, we opened our own clinic with the sole purpose of helping people feel better, look better, and live healthier without the use of medication. We evolved over the years to focus on nutrition and weight loss through detoxification, to reverse the very common metabolic syndrome that is behind so much illness in the U.S. We developed a specific liver detox system to eliminate toxins and promote healthy fat metabolism for increased energy. More importantly, we helped clients learn how to recognize, prepare, and eat real food, not the over-processed, mass-marketed, chemicalized products that pass for food in grocery stores and fast-food joints.

Fresh nutritious food as a way of life is what I teach my patients, to deter the need for hospitals, doctors and medication. Of course, we need modern medical technology to deal with acute health challenges like heart attacks, severe traumas, or debilitating infections. Surgery may be the only option for appendicitis or a brain tumor, angioplasty for a clogged artery, or dialysis for failing kidneys. Infections may require a dose of antibiotics, and an asthma attack will require steroids and breathing therapies.

There is a place in medical practice for such interventions, but whole foods as a way of life can help prevent and reverse many illnesses. Heart disease, diabetes, obesity, cancers, chronic fatigue, chronic pain, and high blood pressure can all be prevented in large part by strengthening our immune system with real, natural foods. Thank God!

If cell phones can be updated almost yearly, we are long overdue for a revision of our society's "healthware." It's time that the old programming of bad food and habitual meds gets replaced with updates on whole-foods nutrition and healthy lifestyles. Download vegetables and fruits, install good fats and organic proteins, and you will have the most powerful healthware around. While you're at it, send the processed foods, sugar-heavy snacks, and diet drinks to your trash-cache. Chances are your medications will also end up being deleted.

Imagine living in a world where the foods we consume every day actually caused many of our chronic ailments. Wait a minute; you don't have to imagine that world because we *do* live in it — a world where processed foods, GMOs, hormones, pesticides, preservatives and other assorted chemicals have invaded our foods and bodies, resulting in a modern plague of chronic conditions that no one should have to live with. If you want to know WTF is really wrong with our health, and what you can do about it, read on....

---

1. See US News & World Report, 9/27/16: *https://health.usnews.com/ health-news/patient-advice/articles/2016-09-27/the-danger-in- taking-prescribed-medications*

FOOD FOR THOUGHT

CHAPTER 1

Health is a Mindset

Let's stop fucking around.
This is the mindset that I have adopted over the years for myself, and imparted (with smiles) to my patients, friends, and family who want to become healthier and happier. As a physician for 26 years, I've concluded that health begins and ends in our heads. Period. Our mindset is the blueprint of our lives for better or worse, positive or negative, toxic or healthy. By and large, the prevailing mindset of the modern world has replaced good with greed, nutrition with poison, whole foods with pharmaceutical drugs, healing with chronic disease, prevention with profits, and awareness with ignorance. When it comes to the state of our modern health, we have eroded into a generation of degeneration.

We are all in this together in a messy world that challenges our health, happiness and laughter. Change for the better is imperative for our health and our children's health. We need a sustainable way of living to promote prevention of disease, and to live a long, high-quality life. How do we become healthier, and smile and laugh more, under these circumstances? We start by changing our minds.

What is in your mind is your life. I've noticed a distinct pattern among the thousands of patients that I've seen: The ones who never seemed to get better, or improved only slightly, had in their mind the idea that they were sick, and weren't changing that idea. They would come to see me again and again because they couldn't see themselves as healthy and strong. Many had complaints of headaches, stomach aches, chest aches… aches, aches and more aches (*ay mi dolor, mi dolor,* as my Spanish-speaking patients would say). These complaints were real but the frequency was unnatural; it's as if many thought they were going to be sick before they actually were. I had a great aunt who would take aspirin because she knew that she was going to have a headache in two days!

If health was a menu, many people would pick poisons to live on — poisons like choosing to perpetually complain, never wanting to get better, enjoying the attention of being sick (everyone has one of these in their family), staying at a miserable job, or hanging on to a toxic relationship. Sometimes when I worked in family practice at Kaiser, I would write on a prescription pad "stat divorce" — as in *immediate removal of spouse* — so that some patients could understand why they always had the same abdominal issues, year-round flu-like symptoms, or other forms of chronic misery. *Leave your damn job,* I might say to another, *and your headaches will stop.* I left my own job in medicine and felt a whole lot better. I don't know if that patient ever got a divorce, but it sure would've been more effective than any antacid.

Your choices from the menu of life can make all the difference. Your desire to be healthier begins with your thoughts. Pay attention to family and friends and yourself to see how thoughts — translated into speech, body language, and attitude — affect a person for good or ill. It's no coincidence that people who find a lot to complain about also tend to complain of chronic ailments. Of course, we get upset and angry and frustrated about daily life. But if we make the connection between the amount of toxic stuff in our head with the sickness or weakness that it brings to our body, then we can begin to make better choices. I learned this firsthand, which helped me deal with being fat and tired with terrible cholesterol levels.

Where I come from

For many years I have been searching for truth and balance in healing — not just the prevention of disease, but the preservation of a high quality of life. This book is the record of my journey of practical enlightenment, a way to share my thoughts and observations on taking responsibility for your own health transformation by empowering you with laughter, peace, and an occasional doughnut.

Growing up in East Los Angeles posed many challenges, including poverty, gang violence and intimidation, limited resources in public education, and the general stigma of failure in the community. Graduation from high school was daunting enough for students in Boyle Heights, acceptance to college and completing a four-year degree even rarer. But these odds never discouraged me, for I had always sensed that I had a destiny of service. I didn't allow the circumstances of my environment to become deterrents. In a way, I rebelled against my inheritance. I was a rebel with a cause.

I was self-conscious as a kid, wearing glasses before I

started school, and a bit chubby. I was studious, shy, and socially awkward. I couldn't say that I fit into any particular social group in elementary school, but teachers noticed that I read well and had me tested for 'gifted' status. I passed the examinations and was promoted to third grade after finishing the first grade. As if things weren't awkward enough, now I was placed in a class with older kids, while I was the same uber-shy bookworm. Throughout my life, I would find myself in some kind of uncomfortable circumstances that contributed to becoming a maverick.

Getting through the perils of gang violence in the neighborhood was a challenge I was able to circumvent by being focused and making it a point to stay out of harm's way. I had friends straddling the line of gang membership, but I kept a safe distance from that part of their life. Many came from broken homes and found a sense of family and recognition in gangs, but at a high price — sometimes their lives. Gang culture is complicated, but ultimately stems from a lack of self-love. Drugs were also present on campus once I entered middle school. Little did I know that becoming a doctor would make me a drug dealer, but one who was legal and licensed: a pusher of pharmaceuticals. I came from a broken community littered with street drugs, only to enter a medical community advocating prescription drugs, and generating a broken community of disease.

I left the graffitied walls of Boyle Heights for the ivy-covered walls of Columbia University in New York City. The year that I graduated high school in 1981, five of us were accepted to Ivy League schools — the first school in east Los Angeles to have that many graduates attending these prestigious schools. I recall our college counselor dissuading us from applying to Stanford, since students from our particular school district weren't accepted there. The stigma loomed large; I went east.

In college, I went rogue as well, studying literature aside from my pre-med classes, instead of the usual science major. This experience was profound for my development as a student and as a person, since my belief is that the arts and other "humanities" are fundamental to our well-being. I continued on to the University of Michigan Medical School, then family practice residency at California Medical Center-USC serving the surrounding poor communities, primarily Latino and African American. I felt I could make a difference helping those who were disadvantaged financially and socially, since this was the world I grew up in.

It was at this point in my life that I encountered one of those uncomfortable moments — really the beginning of years of moments — where I questioned the process of my training. I felt a disconnection between my intention to help and the means by which I was helping. I wondered if this disturbance was telling me something about myself, but off I went to practice medicine anyway. In time, I would confront this disconnection.

The Hypocritical Oath

I did not attend my medical school graduation ceremony, instead going home early to be with family and find a place to settle in for residency training in Los Angeles. An oath is taken at the medical school commencement known as the Hippocratic Oath, which includes the following:

...I will remember that there is art to medicine as well as science and that warmth, sympathy and understanding may outweigh the surgeon's knife or the chemist's drug ... I will prevent disease whenever I can, for prevention is preferable to cure... May I always act so as to preserve the finest traditions of my calling and may I long experience the joy of healing those who seek my help...

This code of practice has eroded over time to such an extent that I often think of it as the "Hypocritical Oath." When we decided to become physicians, in our hearts we had the intent to help people get better. Somewhere along the way this intention got lost. We tend to believe that our treatment options are limited to what we learned in medical school, losing sight of other approaches to healing. We need to open our minds to consider those approaches. I appeal to all physicians to reach within our hearts to find the purity of our original intent, and ask ourselves how we can be better healers instead of automatic prescribers.

The ten-minute cure

Before long, I was a busy physician working at Kaiser Permanente listening to tons of complaints from patients every ten minutes, for that's how our patients were scheduled. We were supposed to fix people in the ten minutes allotted — which is easy enough if you ignore more than half the things they are complaining about. Unfortunately, I wasn't a doctor who could easily ignore so much. On the contrary, I listened and listened... going well beyond the ten-minute mark so that I could provide my patients with the best care I knew, earning the disdain of the office manager.

I soon realized that the more I saw patients, the more they would come back— the same ones, over and over. Many of the patients whom I treated would return frequently, despite the prescriptions I had written them. Some came back because of side effects from medication, or one drug was not working, or more symptoms were developing despite the medicine — there was always something. After a while it all stopped making sense to me. Patients weren't getting rid of their diseases, just living with them. In my mind this was not medicine, being enabled to live with stable disease, rather than being free from disease. I just didn't see many people living a full healthy life of energy and happiness. And that was echoed in my own weight and fatigue.

Until my late thirties, I was eating lots of junk and drinking too much beer. I realized that my health wasn't going to get better unless I changed the way I thought. I changed my mind and my life changed, and it began with saying to myself, "Stop fucking around." I was overweight and tired, with high cholesterol and size XL pants. Needless to say, this was not a personal path I wanted to continue traveling.

At the same time, I'd begun to feel very uneasy about the job I had, questioning the endless prescriptions that led not to healing, but to more and more prescribing. I definitely did not want to take cholesterol-lowering drugs, as common side effects include liver, heart, kidney and muscle tissue injury, increasing the chances of diabetes and a heart attack. So there I was, prescribing medication that I didn't even want to take. Recent studies are showing cholesterol levels that are too low, resulting from medication, can cause rage resulting in suicide or homicide. We need to rethink this approach.

We need to rethink medical education as well. The rigors of training — including countless sleepless nights, the zombie-like conditions of residency, and ongoing education with seminars and conferences — all this leads us to the conclusion that most patients still have to live with chronic disease. Even while still getting my medical education, I often thought: *what kind of bullshit is this?* The mindset of medical school is to focus on disease instead of health, and learn how to prescribe medications that address symptoms rather than nurturing the body. In short, our focus in medicine is the disease process, not the healing process. And there's a reason for that. As Snoop Dogg rapped, "I got my mind on your money and your money on my mind." The fact is that disease care is far more profitable than prevention or health care. This is when the question *WTF is wrong with our health?* entered my mind.

A big part of the problem is the massive pharmaceutical industry. Their propaganda followed me well beyond my medical training, as well-dressed drug reps with shiny shoes and strikingly white teeth took me to dinners, brought me bottles of wine, and treated me to weekend getaways to attend their seminars. This is an effective strategy for encouraging doctors to prescribe their drugs to patients — even drug dealers in the street aren't as pushy!

Look at all the bottles of medication in your home. The average number of drugs prescribed to patients while I was in family practice was four to six. I have a colleague, a practicing physician, who now takes upwards of fifteen medications himself. The business of pharmaceuticals drives the conventional medical model, and we doctors are sometimes the last people to see through the scam. The choice of pills over plants has been the bane of our healthcare for over a century, a mindset of preferring drugs while dismissing the power of food.

Medical education regrettably excludes nutrition in its curriculum. So, we end up graduating with a void in our training and our approach. Some schools may offer an hour or one week, but even that's uncommon. I had zero, zilch, *nada*. By contrast, we are fed two years of pharmacology in medical school. This is the foundation of our medical care system. Patients are placed at a great disadvantage within this medical blind spot. We perform tests that return 'normal' results, yet patients continue to feel unwell and ignored. Co-paying to feel lousy is too high a price to pay; my life experience just happened to wake me up about it.

I finally did stop fucking around, deciding that I was going to change the course of my health by changing my ways of thinking, eating and being. I told myself that from my fortieth birthday onward, I was no longer going to be fat, tired, and at risk for diabetes or a heart attack, regardless of my genes. There was no way I was going to take cholesterol medication and live with the alarming side effects. I was set on giving this gift to myself, and nothing was going to change my mind. The day you really, really want health and happiness, it becomes as easy as picking your favorite doughnut from a box.

Don't bother reading any further...

...if you don't want to be healthy. This book exists to open your eyes to the things that you can do without doctors or medical insurance to greatly impact the health and happiness of you and your family. You can make great progress with one simple rule: More visits to the farmers' market means fewer visits to your doctor. You'll hear me say something like this a number of times, so get used to it:

Be bold and unafraid! Eat some broccoli!

Western medicine has undeniably saved countless lives with medication and surgical intervention, but it has also taken countless lives from the toxic side effects of medication. The current plague of opioid abuse can be traced straight to conventional medical practice.[1] Go see a doctor for your chronic fatigue, obesity, symptoms of diabetes, insomnia, or chronic pain, and the medication you are prescribed may very well have the potential of killing you if taken as directed. We all have to learn to say, "No thank you." Change is imperative for our health and our children.

One day, years after I had left Kaiser, a woman came into my clinic for a weight loss consultation. She was in her early sixties, using a walker since she couldn't support her degenerating knees from carrying excess weight. She was a psychotherapist herself. I spoke to her about lifestyle changes focusing on food, and our clinic's 21-day detox program. I also spoke to her about how to continue on the path to vitality and longevity, after eliminating toxins from her body in a safe supportive manner. The purpose of our program is to show people how they can enjoy delicious wholesome foods all day everyday and easily eat this way the rest of their life experiencing more energy, less pain and less medication. Afterwards, they can indulge in the occasional doughnut.

This patient was given an opportunity to be healthier through food and eliminate years of pain and suffering. She was tired of living with her condition and the pain medication which upset her stomach. And I felt tired just looking at her labor down the hallway! But this therapist told me my program sounded too "inconvenient." She decided to limp away to think about it.

A year later, I saw this woman heading down the sidewalk with a walker, still seriously overweight. I guess she's still thinking about it, but what I'd ask her if I could is: Isn't using a walker, being short of breath, and in chronic pain *inconvenient*? Yes, change is hard but not changing is usually harder. Once you shift your mindset to the thing you want, that's when the magic happens. Fortunately, more times than not, patients that I have seen at my wellness clinic have chosen to make a change in their lives for the better because they are finally tired of being tired. When you feel much better after just a couple of weeks of cleansing your body, your brain loves it and wants to feel that way for a seriously long time. Shift happens!

If a daily pastrami sandwich is too powerful to give up, then close this book and wait until you are ready to go farther. My wife used to smoke cigarettes and tried her best to hide this from me. Faint smells of half smoked cigarettes in the car or mild cigarette breath when I kissed her would piss me off to no end. But when our daughter was born she had to choose. My wife didn't smoke during the pregnancy, nor for sometime after Amelie was born. But the habit did come back. In time, she realized she was putting the three of us at risk, not just herself. She found a hypnotist who treated her effectively, but the change also had to do with Teresa deciding it was time to quit — no more fucking around. Change your mind, change your life.

If a person constantly ruminates on being sick or tired, this negative thought process generally will result in compromised health. My advice to negative thinkers is to heal their attitude in two steps: first, catch yourself thinking redundant, pessimistic thoughts; second, replace these feelings with anything that makes you smile or laugh. For instance: focus on feeling energetic and healthy to 'lighten' the burden on your immune system. Negative thoughts correlate with negative behaviors, perpetuating any ongoing health issues. That can become an unrelenting melodrama that's difficult to escape.

It's no joke that laughter is critical to better health, pun intended. I've actually prescribed watching comedies to patients, just to get them to laugh. Another way to crawl out of a rut is to help someone, whether by tutoring, volunteering, doing a good deed, or simply listening to someone about their interests or issues. Connecting with people and perhaps putting a smile on someone's face takes you to a higher place of being. Nourish your mind with creative endeavors like singing, painting, playing music, working on your culinary skills or taking a class. Remember a lighter mind is a healthier person.

Yogi Berra, a very dead former baseball player, once said that baseball is 90% mental, and the other 50% is physical. With my awesome math skills, I'd say that good health is

80% mental and 20% physical. We don't say "this thought is giving me a cold" or "that thought is killing my back" — although that's probably not far from the truth. At the very least, if you do suffer from any chronic pain, fatigue, excessive weight or diabetes, or any other ailment, you can start on the road to better health by learning to start flushing your mind of toxic thoughts, because they'll keep you hooked on toxic foods.

It all comes down to your decision: you have to choose to be well. It's not up to your doctor. In my years at Kaiser, I would jokingly tell my patients to tear their membership cards in half and throw them away, if they really wanted to be healthier. That's because I noticed that the more frequently patients visited me, the more they embraced their illness instead of their potential for health — which always starts in our mind.

This book is here to help you flush your mind, body and that thing in us called soul, of all the negative things you don't need in your life. Find the rebel in you to be healthy. A good first step is to take a new look at what we consider "normal" in health and diet.

---

1. See Modern Healthcare, "The opioid abuse epidemic: How health-care helped create a crisis": *http://www.modernhealthcare.com/article/20160213/MAGAZINE/302139966*

CHAPTER 2

Abnormal is the New Normal

My father died a few days after New Year's of 2007, after suffering for years. As a son and a doctor, it was doubly difficult to watch him go through his torment. I felt helpless and useless. At the time, I was transitioning into my new career and really didn't know how to approach my dad about his deteriorating health. He would show me all his medications and dose regimens with notes and reminders on his side table. He was encrusted in the disease tradition, and old habits are hard to break. Eventually I realized the best thing that I could do was just be his son — watching ball games on television together, or talking about things that would make him laugh and momentarily forget about his pain.

The last years of my father's life were spent in hospitals and clinics, enduring surgeries and other treatments for prostate cancer, abdominal aneurysms, chronic back pain, and anemia from bleeding ulcers and alcoholism. Tens of thousands of dollars were spent on his last poor-quality years of life. I often wondered what happened to that strong man at the kitchen table when I was a young curious child, staying up late at night as he taught me the geography of Mexico, history, and math, and reminisced about his childhood in New York City.

My dad's decline represents the routine of disease care, with suffering overshadowing living and lots of money going out to the medical industry. Physicians do their best to prescribe the necessary medication for their patients' complaints, since this is the standard of medical education and practice in our country. But just because something is practiced over and over doesn't make it the right way — and definitely not the only way. If you read the side effects of prescription medications, you'll be astounded that these drugs are legal. Anti-depressants can increase the possibility of suicide; cholesterol-lowering medication can increase the risk of kidney, muscle or liver damage; pain medication can cause internal bleeding; anti-inflammatories can increase risks of cancer and life-threatening infections.

All such medications are FDA-approved and many result in "iatrogenic" death. What that means is: *death by medication in appropriate doses.* You've seen the drug commercials with cheerful people running with smiling dogs on a beach, apparently taking their medicine unquestioningly despite the required disclaimers listing all the dangerous consequences.

Abnormal is the new normal. As a whole, our perception of health has become so distorted that we actually believe it's normal to have some chronic medical problem by the time we reach adulthood, if not sooner. You're not in the club unless you are taking some medication for pain, anxiety or fatigue — that is, you're not normal unless something abnormal is going on with your body. Thirty has become the new sixty. This is sheer insanity.

It's as if having some chronic disease is a badge of honor,

earning something for living with pain and disruption. You
hear it all the time:
- "My doctor says that this new drug will improve
  my indigestion."
- "My doctor told me at my last visit that my diabetes
  has never looked better."
- "My doctor prescribed another drug to help my
  obesity since the other one caused heart problems."

Statements like these are now commonly accepted as
signs of progress in medical treatment. But diseases should
never be "improved" or "look better"; the goal should be *to
get rid of them.* The hidden common denominator of all such
scenarios is that a healthy lifestyle is not prescribed the way
drugs are. As physicians, we are not adequately prepared to
prescribe nutrition and lifestyle counseling is not the first
thing on our minds. It is a systemic problem of the medical
approach that desperately needs to be addressed.

This book is offered in the spirit of a team effort between
you, your doctor and myself; I'm not here to oppose all conventional medicine. That being said, I recommend finding
a doctor open to the idea of integrating food as a crucial
factor in your health and well-being. A patient of mine told
me that her endocrinologist scolded her because I wanted
to help reduce her medication, and possibly reverse her diabetes through nutrition and lifestyle change. The endocrinologist told her that the medication was saving her life;
I told her the medication was keeping her sick. That is a big
f'ing difference, no doubt about it.

Let's look at such a case in detail.

Back to Normal:
Reversing Diabetes

A woman in her fifties was referred to me by another patient who had just transformed himself with our fat detox program, losing over fifty pounds in eight weeks. The new patient had insulin-dependent diabetes and was taking metformin and glyburide, along with a statin drug for cholesterol and a blood pressure medication. Diabetic for ten years, she complained of chronic fatigue, chronic weight gain, and chronic frustration, since she'd been getting worse, not better, during her years of treatment.

I explained to her that insulin by its very nature would increase fat production, and the statin drug for cholesterol could increase her insulin resistance, putting her on a path of no return. The oral hypoglycemics she was taking decrease the production of certain B vitamins in the body; B vitamins help remove toxins from the liver. Thus, despite controlling sugar, the ability to remove toxins was diminished. Despite all her medication, she was not going to get better — but she would likely be kept on medication indefinitely. Her doctor had prescribed the traditional drugs for diabetes, adding a cholesterol-lowering drug despite her normal cholesterol levels. It's a reflex for doctors because that's how we are taught to manage diabetes. Actually curing diabetes would require lifestyle changes, and the vast majority of physicians simply don't know how to help anyone with that.

I explained to her that there is really only one disease — inflammation — that goes by many names: arthritis, diabetes, asthma, fibromyalgia, irritable bowel disease, ankylosing spondylitis, obesity, and so on. The key to healing them all is to reduce inflammation, and that's best done by modifying diet, which inevitably means a permanent lifestyle change.

Fortunately, this client was on board with reversing her diabetes this way. I immediately discontinued her cholesterol drug to eliminate its tendency to aggravate diabetes. After one week of detoxification through nutrition and antioxidants in the foods and supplements we initiated, she no longer required insulin. I repeat: no more insulin was needed in the first week, after being on insulin for years! When your body is nourished with real food while eliminating sugars, fructose, gluten, vegetable oils, and the preservatives and pesticides that are prevalent in highly processed foods, the body no longer requires drugs to function as it should. At this point it would actually have been dangerous to inject insulin, since her sugars were normalizing quickly. She dropped seven pounds and felt more energy in her first few days of "food medicine." Over the next weeks she continued to improve until we were able to purge her from all medication; increasingly she realized that the way she'd always eaten was the biggest part of her health problem. She could finally take control of her health and life with the knowledge that she now possessed about food.

Back to Normal:
Reversing Low Libido, Fatigue, and Depression

Another patient presented with chronic fatigue, obesity, insomnia, decreased strength and stamina, decreased libido, and depression — the latter because he had always been strong and athletic but now felt he was deteriorating with age. He was 43 years old — which is not old. His doctor had put him on

Prozac, Ambien, Viagra, and the weight loss pill phentermine.

Anti-depressants have the potential side effects of muscle weakness, decreasing interest in sex, increasing heart rate, and suicidal thinking. Combined with an appetite suppressant, they can also cause accelerated heart rate or heart valve problems, even heart failure. Ambien can be addictive and cause depression. Although he had lost about fifteen pounds on this regimen in two months, he'd experienced palpitations and was resistant to the idea of an anti-depressant. So, we talked about his lifestyle and eating habits to get a clearer understanding of his symptoms and complaints.

I pointed out that many men were experiencing his symptoms due to low testosterone. Low testosterone was a condition chiefly of older men when I was in medical school. But the prevalence of fast foods and exposures to toxins from plastic bottles, heavy metals in personal hygiene products, and pesticides in beer and wine have all added up to chemicals in the body that decrease production of hormones in younger men. The effects include fatigue, belly fat, insomnia, low libido, and depression. Men are becoming emasculated and the medications that are typically prescribed just make things worse. This is abnormal — in fact it's madness — but it's generally regarded as the normal medical approach to lifestyle conditions that could actually be reversed.

We ordered blood tests to determine his hormonal status and overall levels of inflammation. Previously, he was told by his doctor that his testosterone levels were normal for his age (about 300), but I believe that this standard is too low, and should be at least in the 700s. Even though hormones decrease every year after our fourth decade of life, decreases have been accelerated by our toxic lifestyles. I have seen many male patients with low testosterone in their thirties, told by their doctors that it was normal for their age, but it is not. We have accepted deterioration as normal and hormonal imbalance as part of aging without addressing the root causes of decline. And Viagra isn't the answer.

Bio-identical hormones are plant-based and can increase energy, libido, concentration, lean muscle mass and burn fat as well. Prevention of diabetes, high blood pressure, prostate disease, and heart disease in men have also been attributed to its effects. It helps for depression and anxiety, as well as prevention of dementia. I placed this patient on bio-identical testosterone pellets inserted just beneath the skin that last about six months to improve his symptoms. We also discussed helping lose weight with our fat detox program to eliminate toxins and increase his metabolism.

In two months of our detoxification and metabolic reset program along with plant-based testosterone, the patient lost 47 pounds and experienced increased energy and stamina. He no longer needed his medication and felt himself regain his athleticism and confidence of years before. Over time he noticed that his body became leaner and stronger. He now understood the concept of being balanced hormonally and nutritionally, while reducing toxicity.

How did we get into this mess?

Health insurers do not compensate doctors for reversing diabetes or obesity, and certainly not for eliminating medication through nutrition and hormonal balancing. I once submitted a patient's medical treatment to her insurance company to see if I could receive any coverage for the reversal of her weight issues and diabetic condition. I was issued a check for $1.17 — just over a dollar to eliminate disease. I'm sure it cost far more to process the check than it was worth! Most of the time I receive rejection letters from insurers explaining that my treatments aren't recognized as adequate for the conditions treated — even when I get rid of diseases. This is proof positive that so-called "health insurance" is really "disease insurance." The system ensures that you stay sick, rather than getting healthier.

We got into our health care mess because of the prevalence of processed foods, plus the pervasive belief that drugs will keep us healthy as long as we take them for a lifetime — despite harmful side effects and the potential for addiction. The medical community I was nurtured in assumes that patients are resistant to changing their food habits, so why educate them about good nutrition? All that needs to be done is prescribe a drug or two, or three or four, or…

I take hour-long sessions with my patients to educate them on the causes of their diseases, helping them look at their lifestyle choices objectively so that they understand what got them into their health challenges. The option of living without disease motivates people if they are ready to take control of their lives. But they have to be made aware of that option. Many people are not; my dad was one of them.

I had a patient who was told by his doctor that despite his obesity, elevated cholesterol, and chronic fatigue, he was in tip-top shape for a 55-year-old. If that's tip-top, I wouldn't want to know what poor health looks like. Actually, I already know what it looks like, and so do you. But we have lowered the bar so far that being unhealthy is alright, or good enough. This man believed he was healthy until I yelled at him — with love, of course — and in about three months, he transformed into a lean, energized, smiling man. He learned the practical points of nutrition, and years later he is maintaining his new self.

That's what I call normal. His age was irrelevant because it isn't normal to have anything abnormal going on simply because you reach a certain age. As doctors, we are licensed to keep disease in check, but not taught to heal with food. Chronic illness and processed food go hand in hand, and I don't mind yelling about it if that's the only way to get people's attention.

I'll be honest: my first consultation with some chronically ill patients may be experienced as the emotional equivalent of a drive-by shooting. I have to open their eyes somehow to our culture's medical dilemma of focusing on disease maintenance, rather than healing. As disconcerting as it can be for patients, I have to awaken them to the abnormality of what's going on with their health: endless prescriptions that only lead to more prescriptions; detached communication with their doctors, being medicated for their symptoms instead of addressing causes; and believing that they're going to be feeling better soon with yet another drug, but instead experiencing new problems in the form of toxic side effects.

I know just how shocking it can be, and then some. I had to let go of my ego and question my education, training and career, then leave the conventional medical path. I could no longer accept the normalcy of abnormalcy, focusing on disease maintenance by prescribing drugs when actual healing was an option. For a while I was deeply conflicted, feeling the disconnection between my medical education and what I intuitively knew was right. If my medical license revolved around disease, I needed to get centered on healing.

Reversing our modern plagues

Obesity and diabetes have become the new plagues of our time, wiping out the health of both adults and children. Increasingly we regard both as inevitable, unavoidable, and treatable only by medical intervention. Years ago, when I was at Kaiser, I would ask my patients if they wanted to live with diabetes and its consequences, or not. Typically, I got a confused look in response, along with a statement like this: "I thought once I got it, I had to live with it forever." In medical school, we are taught that disease and deterioration is a normal part of life, and any chronic illness stays with you until you die.

While aging is natural, chronic disease doesn't have to be. We could all be like fine red wines, only getting better with age. My experience has convinced me that 80 to 90 percent of disease is preventable if we stop accepting it as a normal process of life. Centuries ago people died from infections, plagues and flus; today we die from toxins in food, the toxic side effects of drugs, and a toxic way of thinking. So, the more toxins that we remove from our life, the less sick we will be. That's the "new normal" understanding of health that I'm trying to help my patients achieve.

One of my clients dropped 16 pounds of toxic weight in two weeks. He went to see his sister, a physician who'd previously "managed" his diabetes, and she noted that his blood pressure and sugar levels had normalized and that he was feeling energetic and looking well, even strutting (see last chapter). She was beside herself, according to my patient, shaking her head in disbelief, and actually told him that his improvements were "not normal" for a diabetic! She truly believed that her brother was supposed to be diabetic for the rest of his life. But he had decided he didn't want to be on medication anymore. That was the decision he had to make, in order to overcome his prior mindset and become healthy. Food became his medicine, as I told him it could be. At first angry and indignant at the changes he was making, his sister eventually realized that it really was better for him to be healthy and happy, instead of staying sick like diabetics were supposed to do.

A similar paradigm shift for all of medicine is imminent. We can no longer sustain the current attitudes of delusion and deterioration, perpetuating treatments that are so misinformed that we believe chronic disease and a poor quality of life is inevitable. The last years of our life should be spent living well, not dying. While death is inevitable, it doesn't have to be managed by the pharmaceutical and processed food industries.

Our shared belief in chronic illness leads directly to inflated hospital costs. It's been estimated that the number of people exposed to unnecessary hospitalization annually is 8.9 million. The total number of iatrogenic deaths is 783,936.[1] It's evident that the mainstream medical model is a leading cause of death and injury in the United States. Why are the rates of obesity, diabetes, and heart disease rising instead of decreasing? If something works, it should stop the problem. There's a little bit of real "food for thought."

The coming health revolution

Most people feel they know how to eat, and believe they don't need to change. Our detox program was designed to have patients feel and see the difference as they progress through a mind-body detoxification process, with unlimited whole food and supplements to restore vitamins, minerals and antioxidants to bodies that have typically been depleted over the years by processed food, chemicals, medication, sugar, alcohol, and caffeine. The toxic build-up over the years causes the body to hold onto more fat that's saturated with toxins. How toxic must your body be if you are holding on to twenty, thirty, fifty or more pounds of unwanted fat? I have a pretty good idea, because that was me years ago.

A health revolution requires a food revolution: a demand for whole foods without harmful chemicals, antibiotics, hormones, or pesticides. Our diorama of bad medicine and bad food can only end in a bad quality of life and premature death.

As the visionary thinker Buckminster Fuller said, "You never change things by fighting the existing reality. To change something, build a new model to make the existing model obsolete." Our medical model is based on the belief that disease is normal, that is, abnormal is normal. If we don't like that model, it's time to create a new model of healing care. That new model begins within us, not without us. The old disease-driven system only becomes obsolete if we create our own health, happiness, and wholeness with a new, health-driven model. Don't wait on that to happen, because nothing changes unless and until you do.

Ask yourself if you are okay with your fatigue, diabetes, obesity, high blood pressure, arthritic joints, insomnia and anxiety, gastritis, and or low libido. Are you happy with endless medication, repeating appointments at the clinic, and a poor quality of life? All of you should be saying, "*WTF Dr Tostado!* Of course we're not, we are ready to start healing!"

Whether specializing in oncology, endocrinology, gastroenterology, or any *ology* for that matter, physicians should know how to help prevent cancer or diabetes, to decrease the necessity for surgeries, and to help children avoid obesity. As doctors, we should all have the same broad perspective on health — how do we heal first, and how do we prevent first, so that cancers, chronic immune problems, and metabolic diseases are forestalled by healthy lifestyle choices.

When we replace disease with healing, fake food with real food, and drugs with nutrition, we're on the way back to "normal." Don't accept chronic ill health and suffering as the normal conditions of life, as pharmaceutical companies and processed food pushers want you to do. To passively accept the greed, recklessness, and carelessness of others is a form of self-destruction. Dare to be healthy and happy. Let's start looking at how you can do that, whatever your starting point may be.

1: "Death by Medicine" report summarized in Science-Based Medicine: *https://sciencebasedmedicine.org/death-by-medicine/*

CHAPTER 3

Changing Your Way of Being

My daughter's birth was my rebirth. I wanted to become a healthier person so I'd be around her for a long time. When Amelie was three, she asked, "Papa, are you going to live forever?" I told her I was working on it.

I was at the nadir of my health when I was a family practice doctor — fat and constantly tired, with high cholesterol. I was only going to get worse, since I wasn't changing anything in my lifestyle. My jeans didn't fit, and impulsive eating plus beer binges weren't helping. We are all con artists when we tell ourselves that we will eventually get around to doing whatever will make us healthier, thinner, more energetic, and more productive. We make resolutions at New Year's, or in advance of our birthday, and then we cheat, lie, and pretend while nothing changes. Eventually I had to decide to give up Lent for Lent — that is, quit the hypocrisy of making temporary changes in order to commit to a real, long-lasting transformation.

I have listened to countless excuses from patients, friends, family, colleagues and myself, all explaining why we couldn't do certain things in order to be healthier and happier. The difficulty is that you have to change more than a habit or two. That's where you might start, but eventually you have to change your way of being. I mentioned the patient who convinced herself that eliminating toxins and eating good, whole foods was just too inconvenient for her — as she walked away with cane in hand, laboring on aching knees. As painful and difficult as it was, she'd grown accustomed to her way of being. Changing that was really what was inconvenient.

Then there was the patient who assured herself that as a business owner she had no time to be healthy. She was always on the go, go, go and really only had time to eat fast food, or junk food from vending machines. She usually ate standing up; talk about eat-and-run! Allowing no time to slow down to be a bit healthier translates to lots of time being sick.

Here are more excuses I've heard, many of them more than once:

- I can't eat fruits and vegetables regularly because I don't like broccoli or apples...
- I'm a police officer and you know we eat dough-nuts and only have time for drive-thru meals...
- I'm Filipino so I only eat white rice and fried pork, no vegetables (that was my wife when we first met)...
- I need my cocktail every night to relax...
- I can only function on a minimum of four cups of coffee per day...

People love their excuses because they justify why they must eat poorly. I lived with my excuses for years, and my wife lived with hers; now we both live without them. That happened because we looked at ourselves honestly and openly, and realized that we wanted to be healthier and happier for our daughter's sake, if not for our own, at first. We all make excuses; it's the tragicomedy of human beings avoiding their own well-being.

Alcoholism runs in my family on my father's side, so I was accustomed to seeing drunken uncles at family get-togethers, singing way off-key to traditional Mexican ballads, sharing their rancid breath as they hugged and kissed me. I didn't think much of it as a child, seeing these antics as amusing — until they weren't. My father was probably the most responsible alcoholic I ever knew. His drinking didn't start until he was in his late thirties, and he worked for more than four decades without missing a single day of work. The only time he missed work for a few days was when he was dying from pneumonia complicated by pleurisy. Even his doctor was impressed that he was still alive after that infection. I wouldn't have been born otherwise. You would never see my father stumbling or drunk like some of my other relatives. But his wine glass never went without a refill, and eventually it caught up to his liver and life. This was part of his being, an effortless daily routine.

Eventually I had a difficult heart-to-heart talk with him at the kitchen table — for the first time as a son teaching his father. As awkward as it was to broach the subject, seeing the shame in his eyes, all I wanted for him was to be healthier. But that was the problem. We can't enforce a new way of being for someone else. As sons, daughters, wives, husbands, parents, doctors, or teachers, we cannot change the heart of anyone for them. You might be able to change their mind for a moment, but the reality is that their heart will always determine who they are. If their heart is dedicated to a toxic lifestyle, that will be their way of life until they decide to make a deep change. I couldn't give my dad a 'heart' transplant to make him a healthier person; it was up to him to transform himself... or not.

Finding your deepest motivation

Some patients have asked if I can't just suck out their fat, and get rid of their obesity and high blood pressure that way. In fact, I am trained in the cosmetic procedure called laser lipolysis (a minimally invasive procedure that uses heat from fiber-optic lasers at various wavelengths to melt body fat). But I prefer to start discussions with patients about their eating habits, and how those may be related to chronic ailments and the appearance issues related to them. Yes, you can get some temporary changes working on the outside, but nothing is changing for real until it comes from the inside.

Many people get more emotional about their looks than their health. I had a severe case of acne in my adolescent years, which made me self-conscious and jealous of clear-skinned friends. So I completely understand wanting to look good on the outside. At the time, I didn't realize that my eating habits weren't helping my skin, with all the soda, sugar, and junk carbs feeding the acne bacteria. Had I known that my face could have improved by working from the inside, I would have saved tons of money on pimple medication that really didn't work anyway, and saved my sense of self-worth in the process. I have seen many patients transform in front of me by starting changes in their mind that their body follows. This change of mind is powerful because it redefines who you are.

When we get emotional about something, we be it. We put ourselves into it like nothing else — like our children, screaming at a rock concert, shopping for clothes, or binge-watching your favorite shows… anything and everything that gets us going and puts us in a zone, that's our being. When your heart connects you to your being, your mind connects you to your doing.

Being aware means listening to your inner self and taking action on what your intuition is telling you. Being healthy requires listening to the messages that your body is giving you — an upset stomach, constipation, too much or too little weight, fatigue, skin rashes, headaches, allergies, and so on. Then you have to decide how long you're going to wait before you do something about those messages. The key is finding your motivation. It's about getting out of your own way, putting aside your brain's rationalizations to allow your heart to come through — and that's when you can start loving yourself more than that damn sandwich, soda, or doughnut.

I wasn't a person who couldn't wait to have children. I could wait, and wait, and wait… or to put it another way, I was a selfish asshole. One night during my internship I was up at 4:30 am admitting a pediatric patient, and the kind nurse on night shift provided all of the paperwork that I needed, including orders that were standard for the admitting diagnosis to facilitate the whole process. That would let me get back to my bed and sleep a bit before waking up at 5:30 am to round with the medical team. The nurse was kind enough to serve me a cup of coffee. Without raising my head, I pushed the cup aside and grumbled, "I don't drink coffee."

She walked away. But I apologized as I was rounding two hours later — and eventually we married. True story.

When our daughter Amelie was about to be born something happened to me; I could no longer be selfish. I began crossing the emotional bridge to health because she gave me purpose and motivation. Your inspiration could likewise be a loved one, or a desire to get off medication, to stop living with chronic disease, or just to feel more energy. Your motivation has to be deep enough to touch the heart of your being. Don't do it just to fit into a pair of jeans, because that's a motivation that won't last. Choose to revolutionize your quality of life and your quality of laughter.

For years I tried inadequately motivated strategies, including the Maybe-Next-Year Approach, the I'll-Get-To-It Tactic, the Last-Doughnut-For-Sure Method, all for naught. Maybe I would be living with diabetes and obesity today if I'd never been inspired by my daughter. For a long time, I was about a doughnut away from diabetes. But I was fortunate enough to find my inspiration without really looking for it. Goals and plans are fulfilled only when you are emotionally invested at the deepest level. Mike Tyson, the former heavyweight champion boxer, famously said "everyone has a plan until I punch them in the face." You need the heart of a champion to get yourself off the metaphorical canvas, and punch the disease or condition that you don't want to live with in the face. Get emotional! Connect, literally and figuratively.

A Chinese proverb that I share with all of my patients suggests: "To know but not to act is not to know." Inaction can keep us enslaved to a life of chronic disease and hopelessness. Being is not just hoping or planning, it's taking action.

In the immortal words of Elvis Costello: *"Everyday, every-day, everyday I write the book."* You can write the book that you want to live, and you don't need a doctor to co-author it. A life of happiness, free of disease, is a way of being that you choose, not a prescription given to you by me or any other doctor.

Choosing your being

Being is the totality of your existence; it means choosing what to be every waking day. A series of actions over time define who you are. If I eat vegetables as my primary food source I am being a vegetarian. If I'm eating fast foods daily, I am being a junk food addict. The point is for you to choose who you want to be at this moment.

In my early years of medical practice, I was a reflection of the traditional medical environment, being the doctor I was trained to be. I chose to be a family practice doctor treating diabetes, obesity, high blood pressure, depression, thyroid disease, arthritis and infections, the way I was trained. Prescribing medications is the standard way of being a doctor. Years later my instincts revolted against this doctor that I was being — looking and feeling toxic, being tired and overweight. I had chosen a direction that led me into toxic health. But it didn't matter since this was the acceptable way of living, knowing that one day I could just take medication for my declining health.

When my daughter was able to eat 'grown up' food, my wife and I chose to feed her wholesome, organic foods so that she grew up healthy with the mindset of eating this way. Today her favorite foods are cauliflower and salmon.

Her health and love for fresh foods was all based on our wanting to have a healthy child. You create the environment that you wish for you and your family. Perhaps you'll do it just for yourself, so I advise you to be selfish in a good way: Choose to make a life of energy, happiness and confidence through nutritious food choices. The people you care for will be inspired and influenced by your positive mindset. A good selfishness actually becomes selfless and empowering to those around you.

The medical system has a poor habit of labeling patients by their disease: you are a diabetic, a cancer patient, an asthmatic, an obese patient, an arthritic and so on. We accept these labels as our identity, that is, our being. But you are not your disease, unless you choose to be.

The diagnosis given to a patient should be looked at as an opportunity to make adjustments and changes. I once diagnosed a woman with diabetes, then congratulated her. To say the least she looked surprised, so I explained that this diagnosis was giving her a chance at a new way of being. All the years of living a certain way resulted in her development of diabetes. Now she had a choice: she could either live with diabetes the rest of her life, taking the required medication and trying to follow dietary restrictions, or change her lifestyle to start reversing diabetes altogether. The choice was living with a chronic disease or living free from disease. And it just doesn't make sense to live with a chronic disease, knowing that it will get worse over the long term. Diabetes has long-term adverse consequences like heart disease and kidney failure.

She listened to me as I went on about lifestyle, since I

had believed for years that health stemmed from our food choices. She was utterly astonished that a medical doctor had given her a choice of living with diabetes or not. Patients are accustomed to hearing about the standard regimen of medications, blood tests, and follow-ups. Many people believe that their health is destined by genetics, or even by the diagnosis of a physician, not by choice and lifestyle. Genetics don't determine our health, we do. Likewise, a diagnosis doesn't give us our identity or way of being, we do.

Support groups can be useful for education on specific conditions and enabling a helpful community with people who share similar issues. But the goal should be to graduate from that group, free of the condition. If you are part of a weight loss or diabetes group for years, sharing recipes and exercise routines while remaining diabetic or overweight, then the point is missed. If we choose to live with a reversible disease, the point is always missed.

My patient ultimately chose to live without diabetes by changing her lifestyle. If you are tired of being sick and tired, then choose to be something else. Being is not endless analysis, pondering the possibilities, or ruminating. Being means taking action. In all my years as a doctor I've observed that the people who are chronically ill have chosen to be, either willingly or unknowingly. It is not the decision of anyone else to define your health, just you. Not the medical system, your doctors, parents, friends, or colleagues; it's you.

Once we can look at the truth and honestly say to ourselves "I am not healthy because I choose an unhealthy way of life," then and only then can you start to be healthy. Being is following that connection in your heart that says "I want to be _____" (you fill in the blank). Whether you're facing up to a toxic relationship, toxic job, or toxic diet, you have choices to make. Make the relationship better or find a relationship that is nurturing, find work that inspires you, and find foods that are nourishing. I know it's not quick or easy. I lived with toxic thoughts, foods and career for years, until I no longer wanted to stew in my own toxicity.

As doctors, all we can do is give guidance and knowledge but ultimately it falls on your ears. We always over-complicate things, coming up with excuses about why we can't be healthy, why we can't give up alcohol, why we desperately need our sugar fix — excuse after excuse. And this is what keeps us unable to move forward. But once our minds and our bodies are cleaned up through whole foods and less toxic thinking, things become clearer and we can walk through the threshold of change.

I can't convince my patients to do anything. When they tell me that eating real foods and cutting down on junk is inconvenient, I respond by asking: Is living with disease convenient? The obvious answer is a resounding NO! You have to decide what is more convenient for you, and then you will gradually become that person without having to think about it since you will be living it, being it. Choose the broccoli or the beer, the doughnut or the avocado, choose to be the procrastinator with endless excuses or the healthy, happier person. It's up to you!

CHAPTER 4

The Generation of Degeneration

We are living in the generation of degeneration. Despite ever more sophisticated medical technology (and more expensive health care) we are sicker, tireder and definitely fatter than ever before. This makes no sense, none. Except that it makes complete sense when we look at the crap we put in our bodies daily, combined with medications we take for a damn long time, if not a lifetime. Our bodies are breaking down as "medicine" supposedly improves, so maybe it's time to reevaluate and change our approach. Our current health care model is broken, and has left too many people ill and broke. We will either continue to co-pay for disease or invest in our health and happiness.

Many people I see at my clinic are beaten and tired, mentally exhausted and overcome by their conditions, even with health insurance covering regular visits to doctors. It's far wiser to invest in yourself with healthier food, because it's your daily habits that will actually heal you. Deductibles, co-pays, appointments, insurance is all "disease talk." You are insured to remain sick for years as long as you co-pay for your disease, which many do, tragically and unknowingly. Health insurance is a misnomer since time and again healing isn't the end game, but chronic disease is.

In my earlier doctor life, parents of my pediatric patients would tell me that their kids just wanted to eat fast food all the time. Many were obese and overactive. My response was that I didn't realize little kids could drive themselves to these places. Parents need to take the helm and introduce their children to nourishing foods to raise a generation of healthy-minded adults. This is how we begin to regenerate ourselves so that medication is replaced by good food, and doctor appointments are no longer a regularly scheduled part of your life.

"There will be, in the next generation or so, a pharmacological method of making people love their servitude, and producing dictatorship without tears, so to speak, producing a kind of painless concentration camp for entire societies, so that people will in fact have their liberties taken away from them, but will rather enjoy it, because they will be distracted from any desire to rebel by propaganda or brainwashing, or brainwashing enhanced by pharmacological methods. And this seems to be the final revolution." — ALDOUS HUXLEY (1961)

Huxley said this at a medical school before I was born. But you don't have to be brainwashed by a medically approved dependence on medications. I understand the need for medications in certain conditions like organ transplants, trauma, or serious infections where immediate and long-term intervention is necessary. But it's the large percentage of people on chronic medication with chronic, reversible degeneration that I am talking about. Obesity at younger and younger ages, diabetes at younger and younger ages, high blood pressure, chronic fatigue, chronic insomnia, heart disease, cancers. Lifestyle is a major factor with many of these diseases, if not the most important. And people are catching on; many of my patients ask me how they can stop their medications and feel good again. Straight up, many patients are tired of taking drugs and want a healing solution for their disease, not more medication that mutes the symptoms.

A patient of mine got the gold standard $10,000 work-up at Cedars Sinai in Los Angeles before I met him at my clinic. He handed me a tome of studies, tests, CT scans, colonoscopies, and more imaging studies with this conclusion by his doctor: Despite high cholesterol, ever-increasing obesity, and perpetual fatigue, he was normal. Prescriptions for all his conditions had been given as expected. I guess I can't blame doctors anymore because metabolic syndrome — the trifecta of high cholesterol, elevated blood pressure, and obesity — is so commonplace that it has indeed become the "norm."

Disease increasingly appears to be the common denominator that ties us together as human beings. It is regrettable that what connects many of us is toxic and negative, a chasm that separates us from joy, liveliness and smiling. This is how we have declined into the generation of degeneration. But we can evolve into an age of regeneration of health, happiness, joy, and strength. This is the world that we can generate if we refuse to accept our corroding bodies.

We have sunk into a world of artificial foods, artificial medicine, and artificial environments where we are closed off from what nature has provided in abundance. Children's obesity has risen to alarming levels due to poor nutrition from fast foods and snack foods filled with preservatives, fructose, and corn syrup. All this leads to liver inflammation, poor sugar metabolism and obesity, resulting in metabolic syndromes like diabetes type 2 (which used to be called "adult onset diabetes.") Young men in their 20s and 30s are experiencing low testosterone levels from endocrine-destructive chemicals in pesticides and household products, heavy metals, and hormones plus antibiotics in our foods. Men are losing masculinity with more body fat accumulation, male breasts, decreased energy, decreased interest in sex, or erectile dysfunction in their 30's. ADHD is diagnosed in both children and adults in profound numbers, largely caused by artificial stimulants in sugar-laden breakfast cereals and fructose-filled soft drinks.

This is the wasteland of modern food and medicine generated by pursuing profit over humanity and health. We need to rely on our common sense and intuition to do what is better for ourselves and our children to sustain a healthy consciousness. If we can reshape this disempowering and dispiriting landscape that brings deprivation and despair to our mind and body, then there is real hope for the present and next generations.

Why would anyone be enthusiastic about taking the next best pill, when not having to take a pill at all is the best thing we can do for our body? What I teach my patients is that not having to take a pill to sleep, control diabetes, lose weight, decrease pain, or lessen the side effects of other pills is the best kind of medicine. Eating foods that heal and supplements that strengthen our physiology is the way to live unshackled by chronic disease, with no need for pills at all. There's no need to accept disease as part of getting old, or settle for believing that breaking down, feeling tired, and taking medication daily is the way to go.

Television commercials would have us believe that it's hip and cool to live with diabetes, obesity, or chronic pain because there is a pharmaceutical available by prescription to keep your disease in check while you skip, dance, or play croquet. We need to refuse this notion that it's natural to live with disease the rest of your life. Most disease is not a consequence of aging but of lifestyle. If you could choose a lifestyle to prevent disease, would it be the way you are living now? To go forward we need to go back to eating fresh foods and enjoying the outdoors as our ancestors once did. Aging and dying are inevitable, but not the poor quality of modern-day life.

Health begins by loving yourself more than your doctor, or doughnuts. I know; I loved doughnuts. That's when my weight was at its highest, and I have a genetic propensity for diabetes. I had an uncle who would put sugar on his candy bars, and died a horrible death from diabetes. To sound like a broken record: you are what you eat, and you become your environment. I truly reflected my environment while working at Kaiser, unaware of the power of nutrition and believing that medication made us healthier. After a few years of working as a family practice doctor, I started admonishing patients for frequently making doctor appointments for chronic ailments. I saw them perpetuating a vicious cycle of illness, more prescriptions, and more illness.

When I left family practice and switched to what I'm

doing now, I began reversing my patients' diabetes, high blood pressure, high cholesterol, obesity, chronic pain, chronic fatigue, chronic anger, and insomnia without prescribing a single drug. What is the purpose of treating symptoms with a constant cycle of drugs while you remain ill and unhappy? You are then investing in your disease, not your health.

Many of my patients fear that their doctor will scold them for not taking their medication, despite having been healed by an alternative approach. Doctors do tend to scold patients for non-compliance. Some doctors have resisted my method, but others have collaborated with me to get their patients off medication. There is an increasing number of physicians who are beginning to see how lifestyle changes can complement their patient care.

Although I am a physician who has come to be anti-antibiotic and pro-probiotic, I understand that our medical system helps tremendously with emergency care and tertiary care, interventions that are lifesaving in matters of life and death. Antibiotics can serve a purpose in the short term, and so can insulin or blood pressure medicine. But prescription drugs should serve only as a bridge until we can restore and nourish health to a sick body. Then let food take over from there, and medication will no longer be needed. Medicide (I made up this word) is what's really going on when we take one prescribed medication after another, most of them with detrimental side effects, all in the name of treating disease.

Doctors and patients can work as a team instead to make choices that heal the body, prevent disease, and create happiness. There are no side effects from broccoli, but there are tons of side effects from medication; just read the labels. The message from the pharmaceutical companies can be powerful: It's okay to be obese, it's okay to have a chronic illness, it's okay to live with diabetes or chronic pain — as long as you take their drugs for the rest of your life. Is this okay with you? I sure hope not.

Living well lifelong

Many of us have had grandparents or great-grandparents living productive, vital lives, walking upright into old age, then passing quietly in their sleep. I think the food from a pre-processed era had a lot to do with it. Death was the end of a healthy fruitful life, not prolonged suffering like my father's. For years, my father and relatives complained of ailments and taking their medication. Family gatherings were filled with stories of surgeries, cancers, stomach problems, and ongoing pain. Not what I'd call the joy of living. Dying peacefully in your sleep at a ripe old age is a worthwhile goal; we should all have a grin on our last day after living a fulfilling life.

Every day, I'm telling my patients to make their eating habits an 80/20 proposition. Eat wholesome foods 80 percent of the time, and leave 20 percent for your treats. (More about this later.) Most people do the reverse, eating poorly 80 to 90 percent of the time and taking occasional breaks for fresh vegetables or healthy, lean proteins.

Nature has provided everything we need to sustain our health and longevity. Genetically we are engineered to live up to 135 years; the majority of people die at around half this age. But we continue to ignore the powerful plethora of natural food medicine that has been provided for us. My model for health is built on a premise to heal and prevent disease, not encourage maintaining it for the rest of your life.

By contrast, a medical system that is currently driven by a 99% focus on medication and medical intervention, with 1% or less devoted to nutrition, cannot help but maintain disease. Doctors, nurses, chiropractors, acupuncturists, hospitalists, dieticians, therapists — anyone who really gives a damn — need to implement nutrition education as an integral part of health care. This is not the same as recommending yet another weight-loss diet, but developing and teaching a full-on understanding of healing and maintaining health with food. It really is time to stop medical madness and bring food to the forefront of health care.

For those of you who want to regenerate yourselves now, start looking at your grocery lists, focusing on the foods you would find on a farm. Keep the junk (like what they'd feed you in a hospital) to a minimum: jello, cookies, crackers, cold cut sandwiches. (Ketchup is not a vegetable, by the way.) Instead, focus on fruit, vegetables, beans, fresh meats, wild fish, nuts, eggs, avocados. This is how I transformed my health and my body, and it's how you can do the same.

"Surgery is the failure of medicine," wrote the Latin American novelist and physician Gabriel Garcia Marquez. Today, I see the practice of modern medicine as the failure of nutrition. Doctors need to develop the willingness to put the prescription pad down and start handing patients suggested grocery lists. Stop explaining side effects of drugs, and instead teach the positive effects of fruits and vegetables.

How many physicians are prepared to listen to their inner voice of common sense, rather than the pitch of the pharmaceutical rep? This is the mission we all need to join, to help everyone become healthier and create a new wave of prevention, progression and longevity — a generation of regeneration.

FEEDING
THE BODY

CHAPTER 5

Why Jesus Had a Six-Pack

We can be pretty sure that Jesus didn't count calories, but it looks like he had an enviable. straight thug six-pack anyway. Next time you go to church or look at a crucifix, check out those celestial abs. He was goddamn ripped! We know that Jesus had serious stress in his time, but we can assume he ate very cleanly — and he walked a lot getting essential natural exercise. This is probably what enabled him to manage issues of betrayal and persecution that would overwhelm the rest of us… and maintain his six-pack at the same time.

Our health would be a lot better if we were more Christ-like about food and exercise. If all the weight loss programs and fad diets available to us really worked, why are 70% of Americans overweight (and 30-35% clinically obese?) We are getting fatter as we count calories, assign points to pizza slices and doughnuts, and drink diet soda. That's half-baked thinking. Diet programs are based on how people like to indulge in sweets, breads, and pizza, so they offer these same foods in smaller portions rather than teaching people about wholesome foods.

A friend of mine visited me after eating breakfast and lunch at a fast-food chain, then had a banana split to top it all off. He complained of stomach pain and loose stools, only to blame the lettuce in his burger for his abdominal distress! It couldn't have been the breakfast sausage sandwich with cheese, or the mounds of syrup and whipped cream on his ice cream, could it? After all, the lettuce on his burger looked wilted. Seriously?! Poor little lettuce leaf, taking all the blame. People love to make excuses even if it means getting sick and fat. I certainly used to. You cannot become healthy consuming reduced-calorie cupcakes or low-fat pizza or fake butter or diet soda, as the food industry and diet programs would have you believe. It's all hype and hypocrisy.

Rather than reducing your fake-food portions and adding up points, it would serve you much better just to eat more real food. While so-called diet foods and low-fat snacks actually make you fat, real foods give you energy. I know this works because I've watched many of our clinic patients transform their lives by eating real food daily, and smiling all the way. I went through my own transformation years ago when I left Kaiser weighing 240, eventually becoming lean and energetic with normal blood tests. Healing happens with real food.

In this regard, modern man has nothing on our Cro-Magnon and Neanderthal brothers of eons ago, eating whatever was growing wild at the time along with any animal protein they could hunt down. They had the organic, natural food thing down! To progress, we can learn from these ancient self-taught nutritionists.

Since the emergence of chemicals in our foods over the last fifty years, we have overwhelmed our bodies like no other time in history. What we are seeing is an adaptation of our bodies to toxins over a span of years, meaning that we become fatter and weaker. We have also become carboholics, increasing blood sugar and insulin that produce body fat (which, by the way, tends to store the chemicals we absorb).

To compensate, some of us develop an almost religious belief in exercise. Exercise shouldn't be an obligation, but an activity that brings you pleasure. Too many people have gym memberships and never use them. I have many patients who do boot camp, Zumba classes, and weight training, yet still struggle with their weight and health. That happens when they are not giving their bodies the foods needed to supply the energy and nutrition to encourage fat metabolism and muscle preservation. Why work out madly only to put low quality foods in your body? Real foods daily will increase the potential benefits of exercise, improve your health, and make you look better, pure and simple.

In fact, it's better not to think of "exercise" and instead consistently pursue some activity that you like: walking, dancing, hiking, hitting tennis balls, swimming, ping pong, rock wall climbing, Tai chi… whatever. Find your "movement passion" so that it becomes a part of your routine rather than forcing an exercise that you end up resenting, then doing nothing at all. If you enjoy going to a gym or getting yelled at by a boot camp instructor, by all means indulge yourself! I encourage outdoor activities to connect with nature since we spend the majority of our time indoors where we cannot activate the best source of vitamin D, the sun.

But if you really hate all forms of exercise, then just eat better! Despite exercising years ago, I didn't notice much difference with my fleshy body. That's because I would eat out regularly, consuming pasta, fried rice, breaded anything, burgers, and processed foods from the market. Once my foods changed, I changed. I am not at all against exercise, but many people are under the impression that a gym membership gives them a pass on food choices. Before or after a workout, people will load up on carbs to "burn them off" — but it's actually pretty hard to burn off pizzas on a regular basis. Bad foods lead to broken bodies, and that's all there is to it.

The importance of Vitamin D
(and getting the 'F' outside to get some 'D'!)

Everyone is low in Vitamin D until proven otherwise… and this has serious consequences, like osteoporosis, bone fractures, dementia, neurological deterioration like multiple sclerosis, and autoimmune disease. Vitamin D is essentially a hormone, once converted in our skin from exposure to the sun, and is responsible for multiple functions from neurotransmission in the brain to calcium balancing in our blood and gut to ensure strong bones and normal cell function. Only the D3 form of supplemental vitamin D is worthwhile for its absorption and bioavailability. Egg yolks, wild mushrooms, fatty fish like salmon, herring and sardines, cheese and liver are foods that contain vitamin D. But the best bet is to get some sun as often as possible — which may require that you stop lurking behind computers, and sitting for hours on the couch absorbing only the light from your TV or smartphone.

In my practice over the years, I've observed that people generally have about half the levels of Vitamin D they should have to be healthy. Hardly anyone connects this widespread chronic shortage to the fact that natural physical activity is increasingly being replaced by virtual experiences with no connection to nature. We need to be conscious of our "e-behavior" so that we don't e-liminate all our healthy connections to the natural world. A digital world is a passive world. Being naturally active is essential to good health, so it's good to regularly disconnect from all your so-called smart devices and spend time in a park, on the beach, or following a trail to absorb sun and fresh air. Take it e-asy!

The gut bone is connected to the brain bone

Most everyone is familiar with the expressions "gut feeling" or "intestinal fortitude." In fact, a significant physiological connection exists between our intestines and the brain. The vagus nerve ties the brain and gut together in a physical and communicative bond, what you might call a neural information highway. What you put in your gut thus affects what the rest of your body does, including the brain.

A recent study in Ireland placed two sets of mice into a stressful situation to see how each set would respond under stressful conditions. One set of mice were fed lactobacilli, the common bacteria probiotic found in yogurt, and the second set of mice were not given the lactobacilli. The mice were then immersed in a tank of water to see how they would respond. The group that wasn't fed the lactobacilli panicked, and struggled to keep themselves from drowning. The mice that were fed the lactobacilli stayed afloat without any signs of anxiety or stress as they swam in the tank.

The food in our gut influences our mood and behavior;

healthy food can give us a healthier mind, but a toxic body leads to a toxic brain. Brain cells are able to regenerate, so removing foods that injure our body cells and tissues can allow our brains to become healthier.The gut is responsible for the majority of serotonin production, correlated with a more positive mood. Toxins and preservatives can alter normal hormone production, negatively affecting how we function. The fiber available from fruits and vegetables is important to moving our bowels and keeping them clean.

To put it another way, if you don't defecate regularly you are full of shit. No kidding: when I was at Kaiser, radiologists would mark 'FOS' on x-rays of the bowel for many patients with abdominal discomfort. Why were so many patients con-stipated, believing it's normal to poop only two or three times weekly? In a word: Lifestyle. In conventional medicine, prescriptions for stool softeners and laxatives ignore the real issue of food choices and malnourishment. Chronic constipation is a set-up for toxins in the colon, as a mass of waste stuck in the gut spills toxins into the bloodstream, causing physical and emotional distress.

I recall during my residency how people with chronic bowel disease or severe constipation had the option of different types of enemas to help them evacuate. One was called a coffee ground enema, using coffee grounds that would be inserted into the rectum to stimulate a bowel movement. I think I would prefer drinking coffee, not having it shoved up my anus. You can also get a fecal enema, meaning the feces of a healthy person are introduced into your colon. Although this can be an effective treatment, once again, I think I'd rather eat more fruits and vegetables and eliminate the foods that plugged my colon.

Our body is completely interconnected and sends messages good or bad along the intricate highways and byways of our neurological system, with the accompanying responses from our immune and hormonal systems.When our immune system is out of whack it can overreact to a toxin disguised as our own body tissue and cause autoimmune disease, meaning that our bodies attack themselves, leading to the breakdown of organs and tissues over time. Hormones may be depleted or over-produced as a response to toxins in our bodies.

For example, excessive cortisol production from repeated stress can develop over time into chronic fatigue, diabetes, high blood pressure, cancer and obesity, or the decreased production of testosterone. Preservatives preserve the profits of processed-food manufacturers, but do not maintain your health. A lifelong diet of processed foods and their built-in toxins invites disease and decline; a fresh-food diet cultivates optimum immunity and vitality.

The common plague of fatigue

These days, everyone has adrenal fatigue until proven otherwise. So many people suffer from insomnia, chronic fatigue, headaches, and just feeling sick and tired.The adrenal glands are about the size of your forefinger and one sits atop each of your kidneys, meaning we have two. They produce our sex hormones like testosterone, DHEA, progesterone, estrogen and other hormones like epinephrine (adrenaline) and the stress hormone cortisol.

Cortisol increases when we are subjected to external

and internal stresses, inducing the so-called "fight or flight" response common to animals in the wild. As my eighth-grade science book described it:

> A zebra is being chased by a lion, causing changes in the body of the zebra including increased heart rate, increased blood circulation to muscles and brain, decreased digestion and increased output of epinephrine from the adrenal glands to stimulate the excitatory areas of the brain to put the zebra in escape mode. Once the zebra is out of danger the body reverses the excitatory functions to allow the zebra to relax and resume digestion. The overall effect caused an increase in cortisol, which then decreases as the zebra rests in safety.

Unlike the zebra, human beings have a harder time reducing cortisol levels, since stress has become the norm in our daily living. Typical stressors include:

- Waking up early (after 4-5 hours of sleep for many)
- Coffee with sugar, soy milk, caramel syrup, and/or whipped cream (what I call your Basic Crappuccino)
- Cigarette or soda break
- WiFi, WiFi, everywhere WiFi
- Fast food for breakfast, lunch, and/or dinner
- Energy drinks
- Sitting in traffic
- Watching any news channel
- Candy break
- Too much alcohol
- Hours of mindless television
- Waking up without smiling

Too often, our response to the effects of these stressors is a sleeping pill, anxiety pill, anti-depressive pill, smoking cessation pill, diet pill, or diabetes pill. The side effects of these medications are daunting and potentially dangerous. Research is showing that sudden death from cardiac arrest can result from casual use of certain sleeping pills and anti-anxiety drugs. More than casual use is the norm.

Adrenal fatigue results in excessive amounts of cortisol production. While cortisol is naturally high in the morning, all the stressors we encounter or indulge in can prevent cortisol from dropping by midday or evening, as it should under "normal" conditions to allow restful sleep. A dysfunctional lifestyle that relies on caffeine, sugar, and/or nicotine to counter chronically high cortisol levels just makes things worse — not to mention beating our livers to death with nonstop junk food.

Many of my patients will say: *But I exercise!* — and then I have to ask with brutal, loving honesty: "So why are you still fat and tired?" I asked myself that same question many times before I understood why. The answer is that the body will hold onto body fat to insulate us from high concentrations of toxins and cortisol levels. No amount of boot camp, long distance running, weight training, or Zumba will significantly reduce body fat until the root cause is addressed. Fat is a successful protective mechanism to a degree — until long-standing toxic build-up can no longer be sustained by our chronically over-stressed bodies, and we begin to break down. In today's world, our bodies are being toxically challenged and can only adapt for so long.

How to counteract daily stress

- Cut out processed foods, the sooner the better.
- Introduce fresh foods daily, the sooner the better.
- Walk after dinner, walk during lunch hour.
- Eat fats like almonds, walnuts, and avocadoes for energy instead of sugary snacks.
- Drink water and herbal teas.
- Limit coffee consumption to the morning, with green or black tea later in the day.
- Disconnect and get away from the computer, smartphone, or tablet as often as possible.
- Find a physical activity you look forward to, not just "exercise" that you don't.
- Detox your body to cleanse liver twice a year or more.
- Cut out processed foods, the sooner the better (this bears repeating!).

To expedite recovery from stress for my patients, I provide nutritional supplements that support the adrenal glands while having patients eat fresh foods and detox to support their bodies. As cortisol levels start balancing, the brain will receive this information and start lifting its boycott on the thyroid gland to encourage fat burning. Not only is belly fat going to reduce, but sleep will improve, energy levels will increase, sugar cravings diminish, and prevention or reversal of disease can become a reality.

Slow metabolism can result from increased cortisol, since the body is attempting to dilute high levels by allowing fat accumulation around cortisol receptors, primarily in the abdomen. The problem is that we often don't get restorative sleep because all the modern-day stressors wreak havoc on our endocrine system. The vicious cycle of sleepless nights, non-restorative sleep, and a chronically fatigued body repeats day after day, and a poor quality of life is set in motion. No way was Jesus a carboholic… Can you imagine him trying to ascend while obese from toxic cortisol levels? That would weigh heavily on anyone's spirit. But we can all choose the saving grace of a healthier lifestyle.

What we put in our bodies matters

Not so long ago, all food was whole, unadulterated and seasonal. It wasn't until a century ago that industrialized agriculture and chemical food processing began to alter the nutritional landscape. Hormones, pesticides, antibiotics, and a host of preservatives now destroy the inner living core of much of our food supply. The daily nutrients that should supply our bodies with the essential building blocks to grow and thrive now thwart our vitality with disease and imbalance. There is no doubt that fructose, corn syrup, bleached flours, non-organic produce and hormone-treated meats damage our physiology, altering our body chemistry and immunity. The common results include obesity, diabetes, a host of autoimmune diseases, cancers, poor quality of life, and premature death.

What we put in our bodies on a regular basis will inevitably show in our health. If we are consuming fast foods and processed snack foods full of sugar or artificial sweeteners, artificial colors, and synthetic vitamins, then we slowly detach ourselves from what is natural and whole. The closer our food is to nature, the closer we are to vibrant health. Food that is grown organically retains the naturally powerful minerals and vitamins that are part of their innate structure. Animal proteins raised on grasses, fed only what is natural to the animal, will not introduce foreign chemicals into our bodies.

On my thirty-ninth birthday, I eliminated red meat and pork from my diet and began focusing on fish, vegetables, fruit, some supplements, and water. I had always been physically active and ate some healthy foods, but with way too many fast foods and junk foods. If not for jumping out of my family genetic pool with the changes I made, then today I would likely be obese and diabetic. Many of my patients feel that the apple doesn't fall far from the tree — that is, their family trees are rotten and genetically determined diseases are coming no matter what. But we have far more power to prevent disease than we tend to think.

As my father used to say, "*es el acto y no las palabras*" — it's the actions we purposefully take that determine who we are. Our genetic make-up will lie dormant if not triggered by outside influences. By make-up, I am referring to the genes that harbor potential disease in our DNA. This awareness allows you to immediately reboot and reconnect your body to nourishment that supports body function, energy, and prevention of disease. I understand the challenges of preparing meals at home, not having time to cook, or not wanting to bother knowing what is healthy and what isn't. But I assure you that it is much more inconvenient to live with chronic illness and its constant companion, a poor quality of life.

Your body is your best gauge. Listen to it. You can live a long but uncomfortable life ignoring what your body is telling you with allergies, constipation, fatigue, weight gain, rashes, bleeding gums, stomach upset, insomnia, headaches, decreased libido, erection problems, chronic aches, joint pain, and so on. We can choose to ignore these messages, as most people do, and still live a lengthy if difficult life. But why? The easiest thing to do is to say that these symptoms will pass... until they don't. Then what? Your body will adapt by getting fatter and your stress hormones will keep elevating, overworking your adrenal glands until they protest from exhaustion and a disease that you cannot ignore sets in.

Case histories of real change

One patient came to me seeking help only for her weight problem. I ordered specific blood tests that included some genetics and markers of toxicity and inflammation to give her a more comprehensive understanding of her body physiology, a body blueprint. She didn't know she was diabetic until I went over the results with her. She also had severe inflammation and toxicity on her blood evaluation, with low testosterone. She was at high risk of heart disease and cancer.

We talked about her lifestyle including eating habits, physical activity, and family life to understand her eating choices and current health condition. In my old doctor coat, I would have done the standard meds, perhaps mention some exercise, and recommend minor dietary changes. The problem is she would have been subjected to medication indefinitely. Instead, I got her started on our fat detox program. She learned to eliminate processed foods quickly, now that she was aware of the consequences of daily sugars, sodas, breads, and fast foods. They were replaced with plant proteins, fruits, beans, vegetables, clean meats, and good fats. Water and green tea became her fluids during the liver detox phase. We introduced bio-identical testosterone therapy to preserve her muscle, increase energy and fat metabolism. After she completed her entire program we repeated her blood work. There were no more abnormal values. She proved to herself that food selections either encourage disease or prevent it.

By helping herself, this patient's spouse and children were also exposed to the idea of maintaining health with food. At first there was a little defiance from the family: "Why all these vegetables and fruits?" they whined. But defiance gradually gave way to curiosity, then sharing of meals, and finally a healthy diet became the family's way of life. To become such a focal point of inspiration for your family is an act of love.

I have a patient with AS, ankylosing spondylitis, a genetic disease that can cause debilitating lower back stiffening of the spine and pelvic joints with chronic agonizing pain and decreased mobility. Certain bacteria have been associated with the disease, like klebsiella and proteus, that thrive on starches. Changing his diet dramatically reduced his pain and stiffness. At all times, we are either feeding disease or feeding our health. We are more empowered than we think!

A policeman saw me at the clinic complaining of low energy, so I discussed the probability of low testosterone as the issue. He assured me that everything was good in the bedroom. I assured him that low testosterone affects people in many other ways than libido, so we checked his blood and he was shocked at how low his testosterone was. He was fit from his martial arts practice but did eat processed food daily, mostly sandwiches. He also had high blood pressure, another indicator of low testosterone. Policemen and firemen are notorious for having low testosterone at all ages, due to the stresses of their jobs. Policemen love their doughnuts, and firemen are exposed to chemicals while fighting fires that severely distress their hormones. When the policeman's testosterone levels were normalized with bio-identical replacement, both his stamina and mental focus improved.

Our triad for achieving health happiness

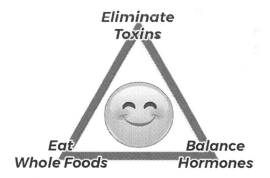

Health happiness is living without pain, chronic disease or fatigue. Often we take health for granted so that when something negative becomes part of our daily living we react with anger or frustration. In our clinic, we take our patients through a triad of treatment that includes our detoxification program, food education, and bio-identical hormone therapy.

What used to be a problem of older people is now prevalent, with men and women in their thirties and forties: low hormone levels. Many people are going through life feeling tired, with difficulty sleeping and losing sexual interest. EDCs (endocrine destructive chemicals) in processed foods are usually the culprits of this hormonal decline earlier in life. Our health is hijacked by bad foods, inadequate hormone levels, and toxins — no wonder we feel like Sisyphus fighting an uphill battle. Most people are not even aware of why they struggle so much. But it is possible to address the most common causes of poor health today, reverse our modern-day diseases, and feel whole again.

I was sitting around a table with friends one night when the issue of how we make health choices became especially clear. One person was diabetic, one had ongoing episodes of throttling gout and high blood pressure, and a third had weight issues with a genetic disposition toward diabetes. I could have easily joined in with the health problems I used to have, had I not made my choice years ago. Living with a diseased body weighs heavily on the mind, making us feel trapped with the foregone conclusion that it is what it is, or these are the cards I've been dealt. But no health condition has to be permanent or destined, just because we believe it is so.

I saw a celebrity-endorsed commercial for a medication to strengthen bones for menopausal women, the side effects of which effects include bone fractures and severe jawbone pain. This is not funny, but so absurd that I burst out laughing at the very idea of promoting a bone-breaking medication to strengthen bones… WTF?

A woman in her late fifties with a history of osteoporosis underwent BHRT (bio-identical hormone therapy) with me for about a year, after which her repeat bone scan showed no signs of her previous diagnosis of osteoporosis. She had been so concerned with her symptoms of low sex drive, fatigue, and memory loss when we first met that she forgot about the potential benefits of BHRT for her bones. She indicated that her increased libido with the hormone therapy proved more critical than she thought — it saved her marriage. The notion of being healthily balanced permeates all aspects of our lives.

Women and men benefit greatly from plant-based hormone therapy for prevention of heart disease, dementia, diabetes, osteoporosis, high blood pressure, and the symptoms that occur with both menopause and andropause (male menopause) like low libido, hot flashes, irritability, chronic pain, aches, fatigue, low confidence, decreased memory and focus. We can improve all this without putting ourselves at risk for bone fractures and blood clots. The thyroid bone is connected to the cortisol bone, which is connected to the testosterone bone, which is connected to the metabolism bone… and so on. Everything is interconnected, and balancing the three components of vital health is the fast track to skipping and whistling through life.

CHAPTER 6

WGF? (What is Good Food?)

So, what did the *red-wine-drinking-fermented-food-mac-robiotic-soy-free-occasional-chocolates-chia-seed-eating-non-GMO-preservative-free-ovo-lacto-plant-based-vego-vegetarian* say to the *paleo-ketogenic-kombucha-drink-ing-gluten-free-Mediterranean-diet-coconut-oil-flaxseed-supplement-taking-lowcarb-once-in-a-while-french-fries-pesca-meat-eating-maniac-aterian?*

"It's all good!"

…and it *is* all good. There is no one recipe for good health other than whole fresh foods, whole fresh foods, whole fresh foods… this should echo in your head as the take-home message of this book. I do not get into the nuances of all the possible healthy diets because you have to do what feels right for you. Eating healthy should never require understanding your basal metabolic rate, or the meta-analysis of carbs to fats to proteins, because all that rapidly becomes too convoluted, too overwhelming, too complicated to deal with… and then you'll quit trying to change. This is why it's much more practical to focus simply on eating fresh, clean, unprocessed foods every day. This is simple and natural to the human way of being. We forgot how to do this only over the last fifty years or so, as the rise of "convenience" foods brought along with it the profound inconvenience of nutrition-related health disorders.

I ask all my patients to rediscover and explore the world of whole, fresh foods to make their own connections between natural nutrition and optimum health. Too many of the convenient and "fast" foods of today increase adrenal stress, making us fat and tired. Anyone can rediscover food that is dense in nutrition and energy-producing, which makes it easier to let go of food that robs energy and stores unneeded fat.

You are a carboholic...

... if, like most people, you eat bad carbs everyday. The bleached flour and sugars in cookies, crackers, pastries, loaf breads, cereals, bagels, and baking mixes have transformed us into carboholic, fat-storing sugar addicts. I was certainly a mad carboholic with my doughnut addiction.

Carboholic bodies store fat because insulin is increased by our pancreas to deal with the excessive intake of sugars. One way to deal with sugars is to convert them to fat. Refined carbohydrates are usually filled with synthetic ingredients, including preservatives, that are foreign to the human body, and the body must also create fat to insulate us from these inglorious bastards. Your body runs on food just like a car runs on fuel; cheaper gas burns less efficiently, leading to less mileage and more engine problems. Running on cheap processed foods and refined carbohydrates, your body's metabolism becomes less efficient, and you get less mileage on the road called life.

Two-thirds of Americans are walking around overweight,

meaning their bodies are fat-storing and energy-poor. Meats laced with hormones and antibiotics are fundamentally changing the digestive environment of many of our bodies. The negative results include imbalances of good and bad bacteria in the intestines, lowering defensive barriers to disease, and blocking absorption of vitamins, minerals, and protein. Pesticides lurking in highly processed foods induce fat storage to hide these toxins in a protective barrier. By the way, that's why dieting does not work: why would the body want to reduce body fat if the fat is protecting us from toxins? Dieting can result in temporary weight loss, but not toxin elimination. Eventually, the body will regain fat to engulf the toxins.

Dieting also teaches you nothing about how to eat better permanently, so old bad habits return quickly. The body is intelligent; all we have to do is feed ourselves real foods, not the stuff in boxes and bags with long lists of chemicals added. I ask all my patients to go to farmers markets and just spend an hour walking around to see and experience living food. It's an epiphany to smell and taste fresh food, unlike the fake stuff that makes us fat and fatigued.

The Good, The Fats, and the Ugly

THE GOOD: Many people ask me, what is health food? My response is that all whole foods are health foods: organically raised, antibiotic-free animal proteins, organic fresh vegetables and fruit, like the ones growing in your backyard, legumes, and natural, unprocessed fats along with fresh, minimally processed herbs and spices. That is quite an extensive list of nutrition possibilities. If you're not eating junk, the best route to your best diet is listening to your body to see how it responds to any whole food that you eat. Omnivore, herbivore, or carnivore really is a matter of choice.

The two healthiest diets in the world are Japanese and Mediterranean. Both cultures focus on seafood — providing lots of omega-3 fats that protect our hearts and brains — fresh vegetables, good fats, and green tea and red wine, respectively. If I had to describe my own way of eating it would be somewhere in the realm of pesca-vega-lamb-once-in-a-while-doughnut-sushi-espresso-fruit-good fats-red wine-o-tarian. I'm vegan by day and omnivore by night. Living healthier doesn't mean being dull or angry about your limited choices in food or life. In fact, it's just the opposite, as you get beyond the boxes of packaged foodstuffs and explore the incredibly diverse variety of fresh, natural foods.

THE FATS: The difference between saturated and unsaturated fats has to do with the chemical bonds between carbon and hydrogen. The more important information you need to know is that that 70% of our brain and nervous system is fat. Yes, we are all fat-heads! We have been misinformed for decades about fat being bad for us — leading to an onslaught of numerous low-fat fads that resulted in the epidemics of obesity, diabetes, and heart disease that we are seeing today. Many people became carboholics to avoid fats, which often means substituting processed or sugar-laden foods for the real stuff.

Consider this: the first balanced meal a naturally fed baby gets is its mother's breast milk, of which half is fat, with the rest being proteins and carbohydrates. The skinny on good fat is that it gives us more energy and reduces hunger. In general, omega 3 and omega 9 fats, when eaten more often than the omega 6 type, decrease inflammation, the root of disease. Omega 3 fats are found in salmon, anchovies, herring, oysters, lamb, chia seeds, and flaxseeds; omega 9 fats include olive oil, avocados, almonds, and walnuts. Omega 6 fats are in beef and chicken, the most commonly eaten animal proteins.

Vegetable oils to avoid include corn, canola, margarine, safflower, soybean, sunflower, cottonseed and peanut (some of these are in common use in fast food restaurants). Oils and fats to cook with include organic butter, ghee, avocado oil, coconut oil, palm oil and grapeseed oil.

THE UGLY: All the processed foods that have replaced whole foods over the decades comprise The Ugly in our daily lives, especially restaurant fast foods, grocery store "convenience" foods, and sodas. If you walk into a super-market, almost everything in the middle aisles in a box, bag, or jar is processed: cereals, peanut butter and jelly, frozen French fries, ice cream, cookies, crackers, chips, breads, pas-tries, pastas, noodles, condiments. Most of these "foods" are laced with synthetic oils and sugars. Synthetic oils are known to lead to heart disease, cancers, and obesity. BHT is a com-mon preservative in breakfast cereals that is associated with liver and kidney disease.

Many of these problematic ingredients and chemicals will not cause significant effects in small doses, but these foods are eaten daily by many people. When was the last time you had just a few french fries or a handful of Captain Crunch? If you have any, you probably have a lot. Food advertising does not encourage us to eat the industry's products sparingly, or in balance with healthier nutrients. All the snack foods so prevalent in this country, including energy and sports drinks endorsed by popular athletes, have no real nutritional value and do nothing but add more preservatives and empty calories to the body.

Also, just because something is labeled as cholesterol-free or fat free means nothing. I've seen cereals marketed as "cholesterol-free" and that's easy to claim, because they are made of grains not animals! My shoes are "fat-free" but it doesn't mean that they are good to eat. (Although I did see an episode of The Three Stooges where Curly and Moe were boiling a shoe to make their soup heartier — putting some sole in the food, I suppose?) You get my drift — marketing is often deceptive, so stick to fresh foods. They will prove their benefits to you in short order.

Is a hamburger and fries really that bad?

In most cases the answer is: *Yes, really bad*. Most fast food burgers are made of meat that is hormone-filled, lousy with antibiotics, and cooked with some synthetic vegetable oil; lettuce, onions and tomatoes that are grown with pesticides; and refined white-flour bread loaded with gluten. The fries will be potatoes from heavily pesticided fields, fried in more synthetic oils known to cause heart disease, and chock-full of sodium, another chemical, not natural sea salt. Then there are the condiments like catsup and mayonnaise, full of sugars and artificial ingredients. Eaten on a regular basis, a burger and fries runs you the risk of heart disease, inflammation, and cancer.

If you make your own burger and fries at home, that can be a different story. Cooking a clean, hormone-free protein with organic toppings like lettuce, onions, tomatoes, avo-cado, catsup (yes organic) and potatoes with sea salt, fried in avocado or grapeseed oil — now we're cooking! Put all this on either gluten-free breads or a lettuce wrap and you are enjoying a real and healthy burger.

Starting by stopping

The foods you eat shouldn't even have ingredient labels, as a general rule. Meat proteins, natural fats, and fresh produce are what they are, so labels aren't necessary — with the exception of organic labeling, that provides some protection against GMOs, hormones, and preservatives. A simple way of looking at whole-food eating is to stick to what our great-grandparents ate, typically from a farm, fresh. Pizza doesn't grow on trees, and soda doesn't come from a well. The "Great-Grandparents Diet" of clean, fresh foods, uncontaminated by toxic additives, is the way to go — although going that way may start with a lot of "stopping' at first:

- Stop shopping in supermarkets for all your groceries.
- Stop buying processed foods from these stores as best you can, meaning everything that comes in boxes and bags with ingredient labels longer than one word.
- Stop eating fast food regularly.
- Stop drinking soda regularly.
- Stop putting sugar in your hot beverages.
- Stop putting sugar on your Captain Crunch —

better yet, stop eating cereal!
- Stop drinking the frappucinos and blended coffees from your favorite coffeehouses — they contain toxic loads of sugar.

Then start mixing up your grocery shopping with farmers markets, natural or organic food stores, and eating from your backyard or community garden. Put more stuff in your grocery cart that has no ingredient labels. For sugar addicts, try stevia or monk fruit sweetener, plant-based calorie-free sugars, raw honey, or coconut sugar to add to coffee or tea.

Switch to organic fruits and vegetables whenever possible; despite the higher price tags, they will cost you much less later in terms of health disorders. 'Wild caught' fish is preferable to 'farm raised' because of the toxins associated with fish that are fed chicken and grains in unnatural environments.(Last I heard, real fish don't eat poultry.)

If plain drinking water bores you, add lemon or lime to make it a flavorful drink with added vitamin C. If you make your own fresh fruit or vegetable juices at home, then that can be part of your water intake. This is a way of 'eating' your water which many people prefer. The more water you give your liver, the more it can flush toxins out of your body, reducing fat and boosting energy.

Why be gluten-free?
Grains and varieties of bread were commonplace in diets dating back 2000 years or more; what was not commonplace was chemically altered agriculture. Amaranth, corn, wheat, and spelt were not farmed on soils saturated with

chemicals to increase crop yields. Traditionally, food did not create disease and weight problems because it wasn't until a century ago that chemicalized agriculture and food processing food became common practices.

Gluten is the protein that gives wheat, rye, and barley elasticity when making bread. Wheat and corn have historically been the easiest crops to grow and harvest with quick turnover. Chemical fertilization has expedited this industrial farming process, with the result of mutating the composition of these foods, making wheat and corn more of a chemical than food. Gluten has mutated to a size which is essentially undigestible; gluten proteins can lodge themselves in our brain and cause inflammation, resulting in neurological disease like dementia and Parkinson's. Dr. David Perlmutter's book *Grain Brain* goes deep into this issue.

Gluten sensitivity is common, and simply eliminating these foods can make you feel so much better. Gluten in the gut has given many people symptoms of bloating, constipation, gas, abdominal pain, rashes, fatigue and forgetfulness. People diagnosed with celiac disease must remove these foods completely, but for most others, eating mostly gluten-free can prevent serious disease and discomfort. Whether you call it naan, croissant, lavash, biscuit, pita, bagel, pan dulce, matzah — no matter how you slice it, it's all bleached flour that tastes fantastic, but in the long run decreases absorption of vitamins and minerals, making us undernourished and susceptible to disease.

There are blood tests to determine if you have gluten sensitivity, but listening to your body is probably more effective. Symptoms of bloating, fatigue, constipation, and abdominal pain may be telling you to avoid glutinous foods; the best way to test is to go without them for at least a few weeks, and see how you feel. Your body is the best barometer.

The following list of alternative flours can help your health. My wife uses these flours for breads, baked goods and pancakes.

- Almond
- Coconut
- Garbanzo bean
- Amaranth
- Buckwheat (actually a grass, not a grain)
- Millet
- Quinoa
- Teff
- Brown rice
- Arrowroot
- Wild Rice

The importance of good food for children

In public schools, most children are fed high-sugar, highly processed meals with low nutritional value; forget about organic fruits and vegetables. At home, many kids are filling up with breakfast cereals loaded with sugar, drinking hormone-filled milk, and then going out for fast food loaded with more sugar and bad fats. It's no wonder that childhood obesity is on the rise.

The good news is that wise food choices at home can help your child grow up healthy and happy. Children mimic their parents, so we need to be eating "grown up food";

otherwise, as the Oompa Loompas sing, "…It's the parents fault!"Strengthening their immune system and optimizing their nutrients will keep their brain and body robust. No parent wants a sickly child, so don't load up your kid with sugar and processed foods that will only reduce the body's chance to fight off illness. Filling up the grocery cart with cereals, chips, sodas, and pop tarts doesn't do them any good. Have your kids participate in their well-being by helping select fruits and vegetables as you go around the market. Make a game by asking for different colors, shapes and sizes to engage them. Giving responsibility to children increases interest and curiosity.

For breakfast, opt for eggs, leftover proteins from dinner, nitrate-free bacon and some fruit. Good fats and proteins keep blood sugars down and give the body longer lasting energy. Most other world cultures prefer proteins and fats for breakfast; sugar-jammed carbs to begin the day is a uniquely American weirdness. Sugars make kids hyperactive and less focused, meaning lots of parent-teacher conferences. We can't let schools, food manufacturers, or industry advertisers dictate our children's health; it is our responsibility and it starts with the food.

A friend of mine is an elementary school teacher who told me of a six-year-old student who was disruptive in class, wouldn't stop talking, wouldn't sit still, couldn't focus on the lessons and constantly interrupted his classmates. My friend asked him how much sugar he had for breakfast before coming to school. His response was laughable, but also sad: he said that he only put two tablespoons of sugar in his coffee! You've heard it all before, but it bears repeating: sugar causes cavities, hyperactivity, less focus and concentration, stomach aches, obesity, allergies, fatigue and poor school performance.

Instead of knowing every kind of sweetened cereal, candy, or junk food on the grocery aisles, raise your children to know of the wonderful variety of whole, natural foods that will feed their growth and minds: pasture raised meats, wild fish, organic vegetables, all fruits, lentils, beans, quinoa, wild rice, brown rice, raw nuts, fats like avocados, coconut oil, eggs, olive oil, grass-fed butter, coconut milk, almond milk, fermented foods like Sauerkraut, tempeh, kimchi, garlic, turmeric, sea salt, herbs, fresh chilies, all kinds of seeds...

There is no one diet for growing up healthy, other than whole food eating. Children learn from their parents, so encourage them to eat a variety of fresh foods so that they grow up with this understanding, and a positive, life-affirming connection with real food.

CHAPTER 7

The 80/20 Way to a Sensible Diet

If nothing else, we should all strive to be *balance-a-terians*. I don't care if you are macrobiotic, vegan, paleo, ketogenic, vegetarian, ovo-lacto, pescatarian, high carb or low carb. Those are all choices one is free to make, based on personal tastes and proclivities. Just know that fresh and untainted foods are the way to go.

I'm 6' 2", weigh 205 pounds and eat less food than most people smaller than I am, because of the good fats and proteins that have replaced my carboholic foods of many years ago, like those daily doughnuts and pasta. I don't do this out of "discipline" but because I finally made a choice to feel good and healthy, then discovered the best way to get there. Eating should be something that comes naturally, not something that you are constantly fretting about because it then becomes an imposition, not a practical lifestyle.

If you discipline yourself with any kind of overly restricted diet, you're going to find less joy in eating, and may end up compensating by consuming too much of something in particular simply because it's "allowed." I've met too many vegetarians who are also pizzatarians, and Atkin's eaters who became baconarians. Some vegetarians eat far fewer vegetables than an omnivore like myself, and Paleolithics generally don't realize that too much meat protein can convert to fat and strain the kidneys.

If there is anything that human beings are fond of, it's labeling ourselves! Rather than concerning ourselves with gastronomic preferences and thinking ill of those who eat differently, we all benefit most from whole food eating. Good health is maintained by exploring a wide variety of foods, and having fun with the process. It's not about constantly compensating for something you really like, or replacing bread with vegetables, bacon with grains, or real meals with vegetable juices. The aim is to experience a balanced, creative, and joyful way of eating every day, meaning that you don't have to think about being healthy. Just like you don't think of defecating — you just automatically doo. I don't command or convince my patients to do anything. I do educate them about the power of whole foods, to empower them to make the choice that will liberate them from diabetes, high blood pressure, pain, fatigue, obesity, stress, insomnia, and depression.

Reviewing lab test results of a vegan patient, I noticed that she was low in her omega-3 index, below physiologic normal levels of vitamin D, and low in vitamin B12. Her testosterone levels were also inadequate. In short, her vegan diet wasn't cutting it, despite taking supplements. She had formerly eaten some animal proteins, so I mentioned the possibility of reintroducing fish to increase her vitamins and omega 3 levels to protect her brain and heart. She had been wanting fish for a while, so we discussed salmon and wild caught lake fish as the primary sources.

Dipping into foods outside your preference is okay,

particularly if a chosen restriction is causing a physiologic deficiency or emotional stress. Also, if a food preference leads you toward having to eat processed foods more than whole foods, it's time to reassess your diet. Too much bacon, too much cheese, or too much bread is not a balanced way of eating.

Orthorectic is a word describing people who become obsessed with eating healthy, to the extent that they actually forget what "health" is. The aim is not to analyze or ruminate on every calorie consumed, or determine the organic status of every morsel of food. We human beings have a penchant for over-complicating things and pushing ourselves into extreme behaviors. What we need to do most is learn to listen to our bodies in order to find the right nutritive balance — not perfection. Even on a whole natural foods lifestyle, a doughnut every now and then ain't gonna kill you.

Striking the exercise balance

I saw an Italian patient who loved her pasta, wine, and boot camp classes at 4:35 am. She came to see me about frustration with her weight, despite all her early morning huffing, puffing, and getting yelled at. I looked at her and said, "All the exercise and yelling that you do doesn't seem to be working, because you're still fat." I thought she was going to slug me. I've noticed that you can call someone a jerk or a cheap bastard and not get a flinch in response, but the moment you say to someone that they are fat — even in an appropriate setting like a clinic — you've crossed the line.

Considering all the pathology that generally comes with obesity, we need to start facing the facts about fat. (I avoided doing so for years myself.) I told my Italian patient that the reason her body didn't reflect all her early-morning effort was because she didn't know how to eat. Climbing, calisthenics, and intense aerobics wouldn't burn her body fat if she kept eating pastas and bread and drinking wine all the while. A little was okay, but not as daily habits. (And why does boot camp have to start so damn early?)

My patient completed our fat detox program, and nine weeks later she looked like a boot camp instructor! She realized that her cravings were reduced by eating fats like eggs, avocados, nuts, and meat proteins, giving her more satisfaction and energy. She still enjoys her pasta and wine, but not every day. She still loves getting yelled at 4:45 am, and I still scratch my head about that. But I no longer worry about getting slugged because she's so much happier.

You don't have to completely give up the foods you love, but you do need to shift your focus to energy foods that help you burn body fat instead of storing it. We cannot pretend that being unhealthy and obese is okay because it isn't. When you've been through years of frustration and feeling let down with conventional dieting and exercise, facing the blunt truth is helpful because it gets to the root of the problem. At one time, smoking cigarettes was endorsed by doctors and cowboys on television. But the truth is that cigarettes cause cancer and kill people, which is not okay.

The same goes for commercials today that show overweight people smiling and happy, simply because they're using the latest heavily-advertised medication to maintain their diabetes. Not okay! In recent years, fat bodies have become common because highly processed carbohydrates and sugars have become staples of our daily eating habits. Too many people are essentially addicts wanting and needing more sugar, more fries, more bread, and more soda, making them fatter and sicker because they are not getting effective nutrition.

Diets fail because they don't address the root problem of lifestyle on a permanent basis. If you find yourself dieting all the time, it's because you haven't actually changed the way you eat. If you diet to fit into a pair of jeans or dress, you already know how that's going to end up. Even if you meet your goal, your weight will balloon soon afterward and in a few months, you'll have to start dieting again. Many people diet with sincerity to lose weight and feel better, but end up regaining weight or unable to lose a single pound. This is an agonizing process and can lead people to revolt and revert to bad eating habits.

This happens all the time, and I address such issues with patients daily. I teach body balance through the understanding of how hormones, toxins, and nutrition work together in a positive or negative dynamic affecting our health, weight, and energy. What I never do is prescribe diet pills. You have to do the work of changing your eating habits, and more importantly, you have to want real and permanent change. I did, and I am so happy I made the choice to help myself and others accomplish the same.

Ask yourself if you are okay with fatigue or obesity, diabetes or high blood pressure, arthritis or insomnia, gastritis or low libido. Are you really okay with endless medications, repeated clinic appointments, chronic disease, and a poor quality of life? If you're ready to face WTF is wrong with you, then you're ready to actually start healing. All you have to lose is a prescription or two (or five or six) — and what you have to gain is a healthy, happy life you may have thought was out of reach.

Initially, many of my patients think that a healthy transformation requires boot-camp discipline and the renunciation of fun. Nothing could be farther from the truth. Once immersed in the world of whole foods and the multitude of flavors and diversity, people realize how delicious and rewarding it is, while they lose weight and gain energy. Most people eat the same things day to day with little variety and believe that their eating habits are "good enough," despite feeling lousy. It's human nature to resist change and stick to the "comfort" of eating the way you always have. But you can also find comfort in foods that make you feel better and look damn good. In the long run, I think that's a more comfortable option.

People come to realize how delicious and sustainable this life transformation is with all the spices, herbs, and multi-cultural food experiences available. Transformation is permanent because it is a new way of being. You become physically and mentally aware of your health and are empowered by that awareness. This is the opposite of having ongoing health issues, causing you to feel disempowered by having no control of your health. Transformation becomes a new understanding that your health and wellness begins with the food that you choose to eat. A doctor does not determine your health, nor do your genetics. *You do.*

You can choose this cycle of ill health…

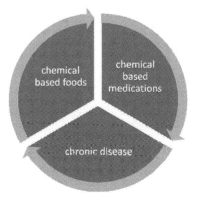

or this cycle of good health…

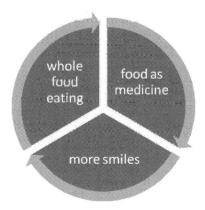

What do you eat if...

…you have a mad hunger and you're at a baseball game, an amusement park, or your aunt and uncle's favorite small-town buffet, where healthy food choices are nonexistent? Then eat whatever looks best, and don't fret. The thought of being enslaved by a healthy diet is contradictory and self-defeating. You can have junk foods without guilt or reproach as long as your "default mode" follows the "80/20" rule: Eat natural, fresh and whole foods 80% of the time, and the remaining 20% is a piece of cake (so to speak).

Hormesis is the concept that a little poison can make us stronger — analogous to letting your kids get a little dirty playing outside in order to develop immunity to microbes in the environment. A cookie here and there, or a piece of farm-raised fish on occasion isn't likely to harm you seriously. The choice to be healthy is not a jail sentence, but a blessing of self-love that you can share with family and friends. Do the best you can in unexpected culinary circumstances — because life will present you with weddings, funerals, family reunions, and parties where you can't control the menu.

On the other hand, a place to visit regularly is your nearest farmers' market. It's not only good for you, it's an opportunity to educate your family. Being outdoors and getting sun for much-need-ed vitamin D puts you in a better mood; you can't possibly have this much joy waiting in line for prescriptions in a drugstore. The more you go to the "farmacy," the less time you'll spend at the pharmacy.

Another healthy, nutritional activity is planting herbs, fruits and vegetables at home. The best fruit I ever tasted in childhood came from our backyard and the neighbor's (yes, I stole plums every once in a while). Creating an herb garden with mint, basil, thyme, oregano, rosemary, sage, and chives can be done in a limited space, providing more flavor for the foods you prepare at home. And if you have room to grow your own vegetables, you'll have the first-hand assurance that they're truly organic. Planting your own produce and watching it grow is both fun and empowering, and is literally good for the whole family.

Whole foods to enjoy

This is not a recipe book (stay tuned!) but I will offer a few general recommendations for preparing fresh, whole, and healthy foods.

SOUPS

Homemade is best using bone broth, chicken broth, beef broth, or fish broth with loads of vegetables and spices. Bone broth has immune building properties to help prevent infections like the flu, or help heal a sick body. Any soup based on boiled bones is densely nutritious and richly flavorful. You can use the bones from pasture-fed animals, adding water, garlic, onions, carrots, celery, and sea salt to make a great soup. If soup is canned, look for organic and preservative-free; you can always add sea salt if necessary.

SALADS

Try different types of mixed greens, lettuces, and vegetables, adding proteins like boiled eggs, grilled chicken, grilled fish, and cooked beans like garbanzo, black, fava, white or black. Seeds and nuts give more crunch and texture. Dressings that are homemade like olive oil mixed with sea salt or lemon give healthy fats to the dish. Balsamic vinegar, apple cider vinegar, or Bragg's aminos give punch to a salad. Seaweed salad is a beautiful thing, in my book. And I'm all about avocados — add this wonderful fat to your salads to get more inflammation-fighting omega 9 in your gullet.

MEATS

Go organic or pasture-raised with all animal proteins. Otherwise you run the risk of being exposed to hormones and antibiotics that stress the liver and can lead to imbalances resulting in disease. In this country, too much emphasis is given to proteins with omega 6 fats that cause inflammation, like chicken and beef, so work on introducing the omega 3 fats. Lamb is high in omega 3 and carnosine, a great combination of heart protection and energy production for the body.

FISH

Stick to fresh, wild caught fish, since farm-raised fish have been associated with high toxin content. In general, lake fish are safer than ocean fish because of the mercury in ocean waters. Fish that are higher in mercury include tuna, marlin, mackerel, shark, and big game fish for the most part. Tilapia and catfish are considered highly toxic since they tend to be farm raised in conditions where they are swimming in their own excrement, and the toxins get transferred to whoever consumes these fish. Wild-caught salmon, cod, halibut, trout, and red snapper are good choices; for the hardcore, sardines and anchovies. Be careful of where your sushi comes from and how it's prepared since raw fish carries the risks of worms and parasites.

VEGETABLES

I always tell my patients to focus on the bitter greens that they hate the least. The more bitter, the better. For example: spinach, kale, asparagus, artichoke, Brussels sprouts, dandelion or chicory, arugula for salads, mustard greens, and beet greens all help clean the liver and decrease body fat. After the greens, the more colorful the vegetables on your plate, the higher the content of vitamins and anti-oxidants to remove toxins from the body. I recommend white or purple cauliflower, onions, eggplant, red and yellow beets, orange, purple potatoes, sweet potatoes, green beans, leeks, okra, nopal (cactus), and seaweed. Note that nightshade vegetables like eggplant, tomatoes, bell peppers, and mushrooms can cause stomach issues or joint pain for some. Listen to your body or get allergy tested to know if these vegetables are affecting you adversely.

Fruit

Go bananas! Berries are high in anti-oxidants, and all fruit has vitamins along with the ability to remove toxins. Mango, papaya, pineapple, kiwi, grapes, strawberries, apples, pears, oranges, peaches, plums to name a few — and organic is always best. What grows on your own fruit trees is easy, and as organic as it gets. Or visit your neighbor's yard at night looking left and right and then make a run for it — or maybe even ask permission.

Beans

Beans are healthy carbohydrates that can be prepared as soups, side dishes, salad ingredients, and snacks. Fresh is the better choice but canned organic beans work if fresh is not available. A simple dish I recommend is garbanzos, cold or heated for a few minutes, then placed in a bowl adding olive oil and sea salt. It is a simple, nutrition-dense dish that keeps you satisfied for hours. Listen to your body since certain beans can be gas-producing for some people. Experiment with all types as I mentioned with the salads.

Offals (*they're not awful*)

Cultures around the world have historically eaten the innards of animals for strength and immunity. Liver, thymus glands, chicken hearts and other organ meats are common foods throughout the globe. Often considered peasant foods, they are quite delicious and happen to be easy on the budget as well. We can benefit from these foods as long as the organs come from organically raised animals. Offals, bones, gizzards, and sweetbreads may not be your first choice, but there's a reason they show up in traditional dishes from around the world.

SNACKS

Most people think snacking is bad, and if it means candy bars or potato chips, they're right. It depends what you snack on. I encourage my patients to use snack time to eat raw nuts, seeds, or fruit, or just drink water or tea. Nuts that I recommend are walnuts, almonds, pistachios, Brazil nuts, and hazel nuts as long as you have no allergies to any of them. Raw is preferable and soaking nuts makes them more easily digestible. Seeds like flax, chia, pumpkin, pepitas can also provide omega 3 fats which are good for heart and brain health.

DRINKS

When I finally decided to be healthy all I drank was water, tea and some red wine on occasion. Coffee has great benefits for fat metabolism, curbing appetite, brain alertness, and regular bowel movements. It's the sugar, cream, or soy and artificial flavors that people put in coffee daily that make it unhealthy and sometimes fattening. But one or two cups of coffee daily with green or black tea, or herbal infusions the rest of the time, can help digestion. Teas have less caffeine than coffee and herbal infusions are caffeine free. If you choose non-caffeinated coffee or tea look for the 'water extracted' designation because that indicates that chemicals are not used to remove caffeine with this process.

A shout-out for coconut oil

Of all the substances called "super-foods," coconut oil is the best. It contains MCT (medium chain triglycerides) which are fats that are easily absorbed and utilized by our bodies and brain as energy. It is anti-microbial so it can help get rid of bacteria, viruses and fungus. Coconut oil has been researched as a food that helps restore memory for people with early-onset Alzheimer's disease. It also benefits the digestive system, burning belly fat and increasing energy levels. Because coconut oil is nutrient-dense it is quite filling; think of it as a slow-burning candle providing energy for hours. You can cook with it, eat it straight, and use it for oil pulling (swishing it in your mouth for ten minutes for teeth and gum health). Coconut oil is a saturated fat, but like real butter and lamb, it's the kind that's beneficial to your health.

Improving your health by half (or more)

In the past years, we have seen amazing transformations of patients who go through our food detoxification. Many people find it daunting when first described, but once they get started the magic begins. Their bodies begin healing from chronic inflammation, chronic pain, chronic indigestion, chronic constipation, chronic weight issues, chronic headaches, chronic fatigue, chronic low libido, chronic anger and even chronic marital problems. We have watched patients reverse diabetes and/or high blood pressure, eliminating the need for medication. People who could never lose weight by dieting have lost ten to thirty pounds of toxic weight in three weeks. We have seen patients eliminate the need for allergy medication, sleeping pills, and pain medication by eating wholesome foods. The path to an unprecedented level of good health is not so much about exercising will-power as it is about awareness and self-love.

The less Cap'n Crunch, the fewer Snickers bars, the less homogenized milk, the less potato chips, the less soda, the less sugar, the less soy, the less gluten, the fewer hotdogs, less bread, and less fast foods, the happier you will be. The more bananas and apples, the more pomegranates, the more figs, the more grapes, the more cherries, the more papayas and mangoes, the more garbanzo beans, the more black beans, the more red beans and fava beans, the more garlic and onions, the more beets, the more celery, the more kale and spinach, the more broccoli, the more asparagus, the more sweet potatoes, the more sea salt, the more cayenne pepper, paprika, and fresh chilies, the more fresh fish, the more grass fed meats and organic eggs, the more good fats like avocados, coconut oil, olive oil, grapeseed oil, sesame oil, the more almonds, the more walnuts and Brazil nuts, the happier you will be. That's because you will be eating energy-producing foods instead of energy-zapping foods, fat-burning foods instead of fat-storing foods, and disease-preventing foods instead of foods that lead to diabetes, gout, fat, fatigue, heart disease, and cancer.

But maybe you're not ready to go that far. If after reading this book, you only drink half the soda, eat half the fast food, eat half the hotdogs, half the pizza, half the pasta, and half the half & half and sugar in your coffee, then you will have decreased the preservatives, sugars, and bad fats in your body by 50%. That's a great start — so I suggest that you keep halving the bad foods until your life becomes whole. I hope you're laughing. I also hope you stop and take notice of your mindset about food and health, in order to begin your own transformation. Take the steps toward healthy change at your pace, but with a clear direction of reducing the foods that have made us all sicker and fatter. Now you are taking control of your own health and your own body. Now you are invested in your healing, instead of inviting disease. *You got this.*

SOUL
FOOD

CHAPTER 8

The Spirit of Good Nutrition

This book focuses on the transformation of health and well-being, primarily through detoxification and dietary changes. But that's not the whole story. I started this book talking about mindset, because we can't make big changes without being willing to change the way we think. In closing I'd like to make just a few comments about how changes in diet and mindset end up changing our whole way of being. For lack of a better term, I'll call that way of being our *spirituality*.

Spirituality doesn't mean shaving your head bald or wearing orange robes. It means finding the innate intelligence and intuition that guides us all toward living better. One aspect of spirituality is learning to listen to your body in order to become healthier. I have certainly experienced intuitive nudges that have pushed me to grow inwardly, with outer changes in behavior.

Jesus had the hardest time convincing people how to be saved, and just trying to share some useful thoughts on forgiveness. Despite his passion, Moses couldn't get many of his fellow Jews to cross the Red Sea to find salvation. Our boy Buddha, suggesting we go inside ourselves to transform to a higher Self, certainly faced some skeptics. I feel a little of these guys' pain when I'm trying to bring patients over the threshold of healing through nutrition, as they put up resistance despite the possibility of having lives less burdened by disease.

Health is about transforming the mind, body and spirit by being aware of our thoughts, being aware of what we put in our stomachs, and being aware of the inner voice that guides us. We can't wait for our medical system to change, so we as individuals and as communities need to explore and strengthen a new mindset of thinking less toxic, eating less toxic, being less toxic and living less toxic.

Some basic spiritual tools

The ancient practice of meditation has been used by many cultures to decrease stress and live with a less congested mind. When your intestines are congested you have what is commonly called constipation. Stuff is stuck and can't get out, making you feel uncomfortable, bloated, gassy, anxious, even angry. That's what happens just at the gut level, so imagine if your brain or heart is congested! All the more reason to release the kind of pent-up waste that fills your head and heart day-to-day. Everything is interconnected. Some of the stress we experience also has physiological roots, coming from the empty processed foods that our bodies must deal with.

Reacquainting with nature is a meditative opportunity because it connects us with a natural force that elevates us. If all we do is take walks in a park or sit on the lawn to look up at the moon and stars, we can still step outside ourselves for a moment to cleanse the emotionally muddled space within ourselves. Overthinking the concept of meditation may just add more congestion and anxiety. That's why I tell my patients to garden, walk, paint, listen to music, listen to birds, take a scenic route home from work, go to the beach, or anything that takes them away from their routines. The point is that you can decrease stress tremendously with simple "alone time," or bonding with nature, without having to chant or sit for hours in a contorted body position.

How we speak also reveals our inner condition. Listen to the words you regularly use and ask yourself if some of them make you feel negative. I don't mind a curse word every now and then (as you've probably noticed) but when it's your entire vocabulary, perhaps it's time to pick up a dictionary. Your words and expressions are a reflection of your inner peace or lack thereof, so give your 'self' a break from excessive f-bombs or words as weapons. Use the other F-words, like fantastic or fabulous or forgive (more on this later). You will find yourself less edgy. Who doesn't like a good F-word?

My wife went to Thailand a few years ago to visit ancient temples and meet a Buddhist monk to teach her to meditate. I had to stay home and work. She spent time with a monk wearing an orange robe with a shaven head. He told Teresa that meditation could be accomplished by simply repeating a single word until you no longer were really aware of thinking of anything else. You could just say *"fig fig fig fig fig...."* as well as anything else. This is the basis of the "mantra," one time-honored method of allowing yourself to escape from your endless thoughts.

Board games with family is another great way to lighten

up the mood and decompress; there can be a meditative quality about checkers or dominoes or Scrabble. I have even advised patients to take up boxing to vent their rage and anger. Laughter, joy and connection with people all create a positive energy in your life. In boxing, you connect with a punch, and in board games you connect with friends and family; either way can bring more positive energy into your life. Whip out the board or tie on the gloves and have a smashing time!

Art is my creative outlet — painting and sketching provide a release that allows another side of my personality to express itself, away from the daily routine of the clinic. I need to remove myself from this routine to let my creativity inform my doctor role with a different energy and perspective. Likewise, you can unleash your own creativity to develop in ways you may have never thought of. We end up placing limits on ourselves, thus feeling restricted or cornered with few choices in life. These mental shackles prevent us from furthering our growth and development. The Buddhists believe that you are either growing or dying day by day. Each time you let go of a limitation, you allow yourself to grow again.

We tend to close down our minds as we grow older, losing the childlike spirit of endless possibility. Plasticity is lost and we become encrusted, walled-off from the possibility of "I can." I regained my "I can" when I left my traditional medical career for the opportunity to teach and help my patients heal through a different mindset. This is why I encourage my patients to find new means of self-expression outside their daily routine. You can always shake the rust off your gray matter, renew faded enthusiasm, and embrace the possibilities of freer and easier life.

The importance of letting go

Voltaire was right when he wrote, "I have chosen to be happy because it is good for my health." Emotional toxins like hatred, resentment, jealousy, judgment, and holding on to the past all erode our spirit. All of us have issues stemming from family dysfunction; I sure did. And some of these issues won't go away on their own. You are the one who needs to detox your spirit and scrape that energy-draining crap off your burdened soul. This is not easy to do, but is well worth the effort and will do wonders for your health. We can keep blaming parents or siblings for our shortcomings and resentments, or... not. We can get off the toxic train that derails our health simply by not focusing on how our family made us imperfect or angry or depressed. This is part of making life choices, a lot like choosing fruit over candy. Which way will you choose — to feel better, or continue to live with emotional toxicity?

Complain, complain, complain results in pain, pain and more pain, both physical and mental. But if you let go of toxic energies that can consume your entire existence, then you can experience a weightlessness of spirit that will actually release physical pain. I've seen both patients and relatives who held onto negativity, causing a buildup of emotional sludge that resulted in chronic illness. Unfortunately, my father went to his grave with anger and resentment over unresolved family conflicts. Those attitudes caused him years of back pain, high blood pressure, an aneurysm, and cancer.

Physical deterioration can be accelerated by holding on to negativity. Toxic emotion and fossilized anger depress our immune system.

That old expression of 'forgive and forget' is some of the best medicine, but a challenging pill to swallow. You will have plenty of opportunities in your lifetime to keep practicing this letting-go of emotional rubbish. We all fight the process, but eventually, if you want to feel better and be better, the walls and barriers around your spirit will start to crumble, releasing your mired mind and hardened heart.

As an historical example, Jesus (the one with the six-pack) forgave and he got light — so light that his dead body rose from death. Now that's an accomplishment! But you don't have to be religious to benefit from forgiveness. If 'milk does the body good' (and I'm not so sure about that) then 'forgiving does the body great'.

During the recession of 2008, my wife and I questioned whether we could survive the revenue droughts and big bills accumulating by the hour. We cursed our situation, feeling the threat of losing everything, maybe even our marriage. But we were also disconnected from inner guidance; the emptiness in our life at that time was a reflection of how barren we were within. The lessons learned from this experience helped us understand what is truly important in our lives: our marriage, our daughter, our love as a family. Stresses will always be there, but digging deep into ourselves was the way to our salvation and peace of mind. Our persistence in restoring our balance made us buoyant, allowed us to grow again, and enabled this book.

Whenever you can, think of all the people for whom

you feel negativity for any reason, from your childhood to the present. Focus briefly on each one, allowing yourself to let them off your "bad" list. Do this exercise frequently to excise your emotional cancer. When you no longer feel like taking a hammer to the knees of certain people, then you'll know your exercises are helping. As you begin to feel relief of any kind, physical or emotional, within yourself, your barriers to well-being are dissolving. When you feel better you treat others better. Haven't you noticed? Put the hammer down, forgive, and give your chaotic soul a rest. You can rest in peace while you are still alive!

The art of healing

I have two patients, a married couple whom I met a few years ago at a seminar focused on reversing diabetes through food and detoxification. We had a lengthy conversation and shared some laughs about the possibilities of living without disease. The wife told me that she'd always felt she didn't have to live with diabetes, but didn't have the information or proper guidance to change her situation. She had been on insulin and a number of other medications for her diabetes, neuropathy (nerve pain and loss of sensation due to nerve damage from diabetes), cholesterol, obesity, and high blood pressure. She impressed upon me her thirty-odd years of seeing a therapist for depression and obsessive-compulsive disorder, added to her poor eating habits, including ravenous encounters with ice cream and cookies.

Her story was typical for chronic disease: the body is weakened, the mind is depressed, and the spirit becomes weary and worn. I don't blame anyone in this situation one bit, for I have been there myself. I assured this kind couple that there indeed was hope and the likelihood that in a few months, she would be living a wholesome life without medication, disease, or despair. As her husband quietly grinned in the background, I told him that his diabetes was a piece of cake considering he was only on two medications! As I presented the realistic possibility of reversing their diabetic conditions within months, they looked a little perplexed and skeptical, considering the many years they had been living with their diseases. No other doctor had ever told them that they could get rid of it all. All those years feeling disempowered and defeated, just like my experience in traditional medicine. I told them that chronic disease is so 20th century. (We won't get fooled again.)

Three months later the husband was no longer diabetic, losing 16 pounds in the process. His blood tests were no longer showing elevated sugars and he enjoyed much more energy. The wife had improved but still had a long way to go… but not much longer. Within six months, she had lost 40 pounds and no longer needed any medication for diabetes, pain or cholesterol.

This wonderful couple was taking painting classes when we met, and encouraged me to continue painting even though I never had classes. We shared thoughts on techniques and mediums and showed each other our works at the clinic. Painting was their soul-cleansing exercise during this entire disease- eliminating journey. We empowered each other through our art and encouraged each other to follow our passions. They embraced my passion for healing and healed themselves.

Finding your personal creative outlet as you heal encourages a life of joy. You may feel trapped and lost in your toxic body right now, but there is time to release the rubbish in your body while you flush the gobbledygook from your mind. I always tell my patients that a clean body is a lean body, but this can only happen if you have a clear mind.

My wife was becoming more serious with cooking after years of reading recipes and chef's techniques, finding her creative meditation almost by mistake. In 2010, she decided to refine her love for cooking by enrolling in culinary school. The kitchen has become her sanctuary, at times spending hours where she loses herself with creativity and love for the meals she prepares for the family or larger gatherings. She fell into her meditative zone without knowing it would be on the kitchen counter. Her meditation was monkfish, not monks; sounds of simmering sauces, not Tibetan chants; smells of roasting herbs, not incense. She is now working on a book about raising healthy children who participate in the creation of the meals. Our daughter has inspired both of us to write books and in the process, find our inner peace.

To be successful at anything, consistency is key. Any form of meditation or healing creative expression is most useful if done consistently. We are all guilty of getting in the way of ourselves, therefore making life much harder than it should be. Learning to let go of myself, not being so consumed by my thoughts and preoccupations, enabled me to achieve much more. Writing this book was on my mind for years, but it took consistent effort to free my mind to let the message flow out of me onto these pages, hopefully inspiring you to take life-changing actions as well. A better you is already in you, you just have to let it come out. Scrape the crap out of your mind as you clean the crap out of your gut, and your life becomes clean, healthy, and happy. There will be more smiles on the way.

CHAPTER 9

A New You, Strutting All Over Town

With all my patients, I try to pass on knowledge that's good for the gut, mind, and soul. I believe our instincts are a direct line to our soul because it tells us what is better and what is potentially harmful for us. I am a huge advocate of nurturing our souls, whether it's playing that favorite Queen song, taking a walk, or exercising our creativity, anything that can pull us toward our imagination and inspiration.

You can eat all-organic food, but if you are overwhelmed by your own negative thoughts and consumed by stress you won't be healthy. Likewise, eating fast food regularly while exercising daily will waste your gym membership. Consistently feeling better and preventing or healing disease requires being aware of the connections between food, physical activity, mental calm and spiritual health. Each feeds off the other in a positive way. Better food gives you more strength and energy for activity; activity increases blood flow and oxygen to your brain and other organs; and some form of meditation, even just slow deep breathing as you sit on the toilet, will help you feel centered and serene.

Smile therapy is also worth mentioning. Even if you stare in the mirror and fake it, smiling will increase the production of hormones in your brain that lift your spirits. Smile ten minutes a day or regularly watch comedies to laugh, thus healing toxic thoughts and enhancing your sense of well-being. Infusing humor into our daily mindset is a big part of healing.

I remember admitting a patient for a mild stroke during my internship, taking him through a neurological exam. I was testing his gag reflex by placing a tongue depressor to the back of his throat, which typically makes you want to vomit. And boy, did his gag reflex work, despite his stroke. His dentures flew across the bed and almost hit the wall. We both laughed uproariously, and his denture less smile brought joy to both of us.

Finally, there is something to be said for nothing. Doing nothing sometimes is critical for the decompression of our over-stimulated brains. Even when my wife is relaxing she tends to be overly active, as her thoughts wander and she gets distracted by one thing after another. She is now realizing how important it is to shut down and really turn off. Sounds obvious, but many people find it hard to turn off after a busy work week, and end up using weekends off to plan more things to fill their time. That's not relaxing, at all.

In a past life I must have been an iguana — I can lie on sand, floors, or grass and absorb sun, basking uninterrupted in a state of mindlessness, doing absolutely nothing. Take it from a doctor: this is safe to try at home. Turning off and recharging is vital to your health.

On my canyon hikes, not far from where I live, I love

encountering the smell of lavender, and I can understand why Vincent Van Gogh loved painting in the fields of southern France. By taking in the scents, sounds and beauty of nature a few times a month, your mind will be put at ease without having to resort to Valium or a second martini. It's about getting outside to refresh that mind and brain with air that isn't coming from an AC unit. The closer we are to nature, the closer we are to health.

It's been my observation that when people strut it's a sign of extreme confidence. My goal is to have people strutting all over town. I see patients slump into my clinic depressed and tired, having no awareness that they can transform themselves. It's beautiful to see them strutting down my hallway — after they've transformed from haggard, distraught, frustrated patients to confident, happy people. It's about a food revolution, knowledge revolution, and self-empowerment revolution. The fast track to strutting is getting rid of the shit from the head, stomach and soul!

We are all imperfect human beings, and going after perfection will only exhaust us. Striving for balance in what we think, what we eat, and how we behave is what will calm us, and also help calm the chaotic, toxic world around us. When I'm talking to a patient about being healthy, but he is thinking about how his parents are suffering from chronic pain with a poor quality of life, then there is little reason to wish for a long life. A poor quality of life is normal for many people, so why prolong the agony? "Might as well keep eating the way I like and not change a thing."

This is the teaching opportunity that I have: to dislodge this kind of thinking in my patients and help them replace it with the awareness that changing ritual choices and habits can change their lives for good. And that's true even if they can manage only small adjustments at first, because that's the first step toward a healthy balance. But we need to listen for the higher voice within us, not the nonstop, anxious self-talk that usually blocks everything else out.

Several times, I thought seriously about quitting medical school. I felt discouraged going through a system that felt so detached and dehumanizing. In retrospect, I went through this crucible with a feeling of discontent, trying to find my role. Something kept me going through the maelstrom, not knowing where I was heading. I can now appreciate the hours of sleeplessness, beepers sounding off endlessly, and memorizing thousands of pages from medical texts over the years, which brought me to this moment. Years of sacrifice in labs, libraries and hospitals are behind this little book. All those years, I was reluctant but listened to my truth to get through it all, so that I could eventually define myself as the kind of doctor I want to be, and share my learning with sincerity, candor and humor.

Your intuition is a spiritual message given to you without interference from logical thoughts or knowledge — it just IS. Finding this "ISness" within yourself will guide you to your health and happiness. I felt like crap every time I went out to drink beer all night with friends, until I realized that the time had come to make choices which make me feel less lousy. Likewise, if you feel lousy about your job it means you need a new kind of work, and if you feel lousy about your marriage, it's time to do something about it. Follow your 'ISness' because there is more happiness when you find it, however long that takes.

You create a ritual of habits, a routine, that eventually defines you. You frequent a pub, feeling good about the effects of alcohol and the connection with others that drink like you, creating a ritual. Or, you stop by a bakery or coffee shop each morning before heading off to work for pastry with your coffee, and off you go. Some folks are up at the crack of dawn jogging, or off to spin or yoga class. Many of my patients wonder why they feel tired or haggard or worn out, not realizing the consequences of their rituals. One doughnut, two doughnuts, three doughnuts eventually equals thousands. The same goes for cigarettes, sodas, burgers and fries, or cocktails, until your body breaks.

Transformation begins with the little daily change or shift that, over time, creates a new you. It took me a while to recognize how unhealthy and fat I had become. Obviously, the weekly pitchers of beer and take-out rituals weren't helping me. When I finally did see what I'd become and didn't like how I felt — realizing that my daily routines made me who I was — I needed to start thinking, feeling, and acting differently to become a different person.

The skill of good selfishness

You can't live in peace always wanting to be right. My father was emphatic about being right all the time, to the point where hearing "You're wrong!" would leave a bitter taste in my mouth. Being right all the time means you are trying to control everything in your life. Then, anything that doesn't go according to plan knocks you around, and you end up feeling pissed, aggravated, and impatient instead of peaceful. Always feeling challenged or indignant will over-activate hormones like cortisol and epinephrine, which can spell "heart issues" down the line.

Allowing different perspectives on important issues can bring more balance and harmony to our mindset and hormonal state. No one knows it all, and it serves us better to be open and willing to learn from other perspectives than our own. We can't force others to see things the way we do, but we can be flexible and make peace with our differences, rather than haranguing each other.

I teach my patients what I call "good selfishness." The idea is to set aside some time with no regard for anything else (i.e., family, friends, television, electronic devices) so that you create a boundary between yourself and any stresses of the world. This is not about being a selfish bastard, but about being a self-loving, self-preserving YOU. Giving yourself the rigorous attention you would your child, spouse, or pet, you apply this unconditional love to yourself. It is how you can receive the gift of solitude, peace and calm.

This is critical for your health because it detaches you from the fixed responsibilities and craziness of life and starts you on your way to detoxing your spirit. Demanding this positive selfishness for a few minutes a day is as important as sleep and taking a dump, because you are dumping all the toxins filling your mind and stagnating your spirit. Sleeping deletes stress of the mind, defecating eliminates toxic waste from your body, detaching yourself washes away spiritual toxins. Here are some tips on these real, doable exercises:

Sleep: the best anti-aging medicine around. just as computers go into sleep mode, your brain needs to go into sleep mode. Turn off all wi-fi wherever you sleep, put cell phones on 'airplane mode" and sleep no less than six hours; more is better. There is nothing to be proud of in getting too little sleep. Can't sleep? Check testosterone and estrogen levels, do a liver detox, and stick to green tea for a stimulant.

Dump: More is better. Eliminating toxins from your body is the key to preventing disease. Can't poop? Do a liver cleanse, eat and drink water with fruit and veggies, use coconut oil in coffee or a protein shake daily. High fiber foods are important for healthy elimination.

Detach: Love of self is not to be confused with self-ishness. After all, it's the same unconditional love you give your partner, children, and pets. The more you focus on pre-serving yourself, the more you can be of service and use to your family and loved ones. What's important is that you disconnect and disengage from your head and let your spirit roam free. How? Taking walks, taking a bath, playing a musical instrument, losing yourself in a book or music, or just turning off to do nothing. For those who are overly wired, too connected to the digital world, connect with your thoughts and feelings instead to soothe your spirit.

When you are operating as a high-performance self you don't carry around any junk. Junk comes in the form of foods, negative thoughts, lifetime grudges. Before self-transforma-tion, any kind of fuel seems to be okay. Afterwards, you'll desire and demand high-octane fuel for body, mind, and spirit. This kind of fuel keeps you on the road to being one fierce, healthy motherfucker. You can flush negative thoughts, flush toxic waste, and flush debilitating stress with-out medication, without insurance, without a doctor. It's all free and the benefits are immeasurable. If being healthy is radical, then it's time we bring out that rebel in all of us. You are the one in charge of your health. The potential for optimal performance and happiness is within each one of us—and that means you, my friend. Let's see you strut!

Afterword

I hope this book has helped you see how our mindset influences our being, and understand how we've come to regard abnormal health and dietary conditions as normal. So, what can we do to create a healing trend for this generation of degeneration? It's time to make the truly normal normal again, by creating a mindset of powerful good health based on wholesome nutrition. We must all take responsibility for creating a world where we respect life and help each other understand the consequences of choices that we make. Common sense tells us that our modern healthcare system is broken and needs to be fixed. Through education and food awareness, more doctors can share this vision to make a difference in people's lives and happiness. But we need many more voices and much more education for doctors and patients alike to work together towards a clean and healthy lifestyle. These are the values that I share with my young daughter to help create a more nurturing and nourishing world. I challenge each one of us to contribute to a generation of regeneration through our choices and values. This is the gift that I've happily shared with patients, and now this book gives me the opportunity to share it with every reader to help you live a life of laughter and joy.

— *Roberto Tostado M.D.*

The Benefits of Detoxing

Body purification has been around for thousands of years and has been practiced in many cultures in many different ways. In this modern world, we are constantly exposed to external toxins on a daily basis, through the air we breathe, the water we drink, foods ridden with chemicals, pesticides, preservatives, and prescription drugs. The liver is a powerful organ that functions as the main filter of our body with the capacity to cleanse, filter and remove toxins from our bodies. An overworked liver can affect major functions of our bodies, causing our systems to break down.

After leaving family practice, I focused on my intuition about nutrition being paramount to our wellbeing. As I learned to treat my patients nutritionally I realized how detoxing has become necessary to help prevent and reverse diseases that affect many of us today. Decades ago this wasn't the case since foods then were fresh and organic without having to be labeled as such.

I created the IBODY Transformation Cleanse so that my patients could experience food as their medicine. Despite educating on better food habits, patients would still hit a plateau in their progress. Liver detoxification has truly become a necessity to preserve our health to help prevent and reverse diseases that affect many of us today.

Similar to the air filter of a car, our liver can become over-worked and clogged, causing malfunction and inefficiency. Lack of energy, poor sleep patterns and weight gain result as our inefficient liver bury toxins into fat that it is incapable of eliminating to protect our body from its harmful effects. We experience a wide range of symptoms that we may attribute to our daily stresses, but actually result from poor liver function. Detox is a fast track to a significantly higher plane of health in a relatively short period of time.

In the first few days of the program patients can usually feel the effects of toxins as they make their way out of the body, experiencing symptoms like aches and fatigue. Within just days patients will begin to feel much more energy, better sleep, clearer skin, improved mental focus, and less body pain. Shedding toxic weight is typical, and can be significant depending on the amount of excess body fat.

I have seen the power of healing with foods over many years of implementing this simple program. The detox program is done over 21 days to allow ample time to remove years of accumulated toxins from the body, while learning how to replace artificial foods with whole foods. It takes at least three weeks to enable people to break bad food habits and create new positive ones that help heal the body and shed excess weight.

This kit has helped my patients begin to reverse diabetes, lose weight, drastically improve digestion, reduce medication, and create smiles. Some patients have been skeptical when I introduce the idea of food as their medicine but the outcomes have surprised even them as it becomes a lifestyle.

Prior to beginning the detox program, one of our patients drank two pots of coffee daily and ate fast food regularly. The first day was unpleasant for him, since he was not allowed to have coffee during the program. Removing any form of stimulant that the body depends on for energy is key to the detoxification process. He experienced a caffeine withdrawal headache and almost quit. However, encouraged by his wife, who also was going through the cleanse, he soldiered through the process and was so grateful that he did. After three weeks, he had lost 25 pounds and came to the realization that the copious amounts of coffee he had been consuming were no longer necessary. His energy was now coming from the foods he was eating, not the caffeine he previously thought was needed for his lack of energy.

It's shocking how many patients realize how much more energy they feel without all the caffeinated drinks that they used prior to the detox. Many discover the joy of regular bowel movements, a flatter stomach, deep refreshing sleep and increased mental focus that come with eating whole foods and resting the liver. The body rapidly adapts to whole foods to transform from a carboholic state to a fat-burning, energy-producing state. A carboholic brain can be quite powerful, but its hold can be broken through the elimination of toxins, and their replacement with dense food nutrients, essential enzymes, vitamins and minerals. It is truly amazing that years of abusing the body with junk food can be reversed in such a short period, and easily maintained as fresh foods replace processed ones.

Another patient in his late fifties introduced himself by telling me that he had his diabetes under control with drugs, had high blood pressure and high cholesterol, also being treated with medication, and experienced fatigue with decreased stamina. Taking "only" five medications by prescription, he insisted that he was doing quite well for his age! I repeated back the problems he had listed, feeling compelled to inform him that he was not, in fact, healthy. But millions of people are on a regimen of various medications, feel fatigued, and are overweight or obese, all the while thinking these conditions are acceptable. This patient was a little surprised that a physician spoke to him so candidly. But he was even more surprised when I told him he could reverse his medical conditions and look better, feel better, and think better utilizing only the healing properties of food.

I put him through our detoxification program to clean his gunk-filled liver. During the 21-day program, he took daily capsules of concentrated organic vegetables and fruit, with all of their inherent vitamins and minerals and essential amino acids that stimulate the liver to commence and support the detoxification process. He also drank a daily greens shake made with cruciferous vegetables, the bitter greens that most people hate (but your liver loves). The beauty is that it tastes nothing like boiled Brussels sprouts; quite the opposite in fact, it's delicious. He was instructed to eat unlimited fruits, vegetables, some brown rice, hearty soups, salads, lentil 'burgers' or lentil 'tacos' with lettuce wraps sea-soned with fresh herbs. The patient was introduced to eating good fats like avocados and cooking with healthy oils such as olive, grapeseed, and coconut. (Organic meat proteins or wild caught fish is introduced after a few days.)

Within weeks, this guy who'd thought he was healthy

with multiple health conditions and medications was now strutting and smiling, thirty pounds lighter with no more abnormal blood sugar, no more high blood pressure, and no medication. He had also learned how to eat, and loves what he eats now. All because he chose to be someone who didn't want to live with chronic illness, instead choosing to live in a way that would prevent disease instead of inviting it. The time frame differs for each patient depending on toxicity levels and disease progression. But weeks to months is realistic for most people, to start turning their conditions around. Compare that to year after year of conventional prescription medications for serious chronic ailments, with no real improvement or endpoint in sight.

Getting sick is a process, so getting well is also a process. But the rewards of choosing to be well far surpass the inconvenience of giving up a few things that make us sick.

A friend of mine, Charles Murray, lived in Japan a few years after completing his law degree to teach English before starting his practice in Los Angeles. He wanted the opportunity to live outside his comfort zone and immerse himself in a different culture. While in Japan, he noticed that over time he lost weight without intentionally trying, and became more energetic. He ate what was available daily like fish, rice and some vegetables, all the while riding a bike to work. The food and exercise became an extension of himself, a lifestyle that resulted in a healthier version of who he was prior to living in Japan. It became a natural way of living and eating the way I encourage patients to live — nothing overcomplicated.

I encourage you to do your own mild version of detox at home with these simple steps. Go an entire week without any prepackaged, processed or fast foods and eat unlimited amounts of the whole foods suggested in this book. Avoid animal proteins during this time to give your liver a break, and allow it to focus on expelling backed-up toxins in your system instead of storing it in your fat. Animal protein requires a lot more work on your liver to digest, so do your best. Avoid alcohol and caffeine. Drink lots of water daily with non-caffeinated herbal teas. Challenge yourself to go a day longer with each succeeding cleanse. This a shortcut to feeling better and it doesn't cost you anything.

When you are ready you can advance to a more formal detox program like our IBODY cleanse. There are other good programs available out there, but make sure that the supplements in any program are whole-food based. For those of you who are on medication just make sure your doctor supervises your progress.

Find your 80/20 and an exercise that you enjoy doing with a regular detox as part of your routine. These positive changes will become your lifestyle and you'll no longer have to think about being healthy, you just will be…as you strut all around town, of course.

For more information, see *www.ibodydetox.com*.

ACKNOWLEDGEMENTS
& INSPIRATIONS

Loads of thank-yous and gratitude are owed for the making of this book that I wrote over six years. My intent was to let people know the truth of how to obtain health through choice and food, partly because I was tired of hearing my voice explaining this over the years to one person at a time. Now I could yell at many people at once! At one point my original manuscript was lost for two years after my computer imploded. Starting over was a blessing in disguise, allowing me to write more from the heart than the head. I thank my wife Teresa for being by me every step of the way in my book and life with her love, endless encouragement and insight on this project so that it reflected all sides of me, my humor, my F-words, frustration, inspiration and honesty. I now look forward to my wife's book on raising a healthy child and family with awesome recipes.

I have dedicated this book to Amelie, but I also thank her for her young wisdom and encouragement to get this book out. As she said to me, "Papa, even if it only changes the life of one person it was worth it."

Thanks to my father, who instilled in me practical values and integrity, and to my mom, turning 90, for believing in me and giving her unconditional love. She lives a healthy life because she eats well, enjoys wine, laughs and listens to me of course.

Thanks to D. Patrick Miller, editor virtuoso, despite my frustrating him countless times with my F-words and unique style of expression. I am forever grateful that Patrick took on this radical book, meant to empower and give practical understanding of health and happiness. I detoxed him and now he struts more. His company name, Fearless Books, rocks — and reflects the reason he took me on.

I also want to thank my musical inspirations while writing this book, including Queen, Freddy Mercury, The Who, and Coltrane. I was also inspired by Rich Rolls book *Finding Ultra*, to continue writing my book on my transformation to help others find theirs. I would like to thank all of my patients for believing in my passion and choosing to become healthy. I thank the readers for giving yourself the possibility of a life filled with strutting and smiles. Thank God for making me the way I am and inspiring me to write.

And lastly, I would like to thank me for writing this damn book while being a husband, a papa, and helping patients become rebels in finding their f'ing health and happiness through food...and a little forgiveness.

I thank you all.

Made in the USA
San Bernardino, CA
31 July 2019